Pediatric Dentistry

Editor

JOEL H. BERG

DENTAL CLINICS OF NORTH AMERICA

www.dental.theclinics.com

January 2013 • Volume 57 • Number 1

Contributors

GUEST EDITOR

JOEL H. BERG, DDS, MS
Dean, Professor, Department of Pediatric Dentistry, Lloyd and Kay Chapman Chair for Oral Health, School of Dentistry, University of Washington, Seattle, Washington; President, American Academy of Pediatric Dentistry, Chicago, Illinois

AUTHORS

JOEL H. BERG, DDS, MS
Dean, Professor, Department of Pediatric Dentistry, Lloyd and Kay Chapman Chair for Oral Health, School of Dentistry, University of Washington, Seattle, Washington; President, American Academy of Pediatric Dentistry, Chicago, Illinois

ISABELLE CHASE, DDS
Director of Pre-doctoral Pediatric Dentistry, Boston Children's Hospital, Instructor of Developmental Biology (Pediatric Dentistry), Harvard School of Dental Medicine, Boston, Massachusetts

NESTOR COHENCA, DDS
Departments of Endodontics and Pediatric Dentistry, School of Dentistry, University of Washington, Seattle, Washington

KEVIN J. DONLY, DDS, MS
Professor and Chair, Department of Developmental Dentistry, Dental School, University of Texas Health Science Center at San Antonio, San Antonio, Texas

JAMES A. HOWARD, DDS
Clinical Assistant Professor, Center for Pediatric Dentistry, School of Dentistry, University of Washington; Chief, Temporomandibular Joint Dysfunction Clinic, Seattle Children's Hospital, Seattle, Washington

ELIZABETH KUTCIPAL, DDS
Oral and Maxillofacial Surgeon, Seattle Children's Hospital; Affiliate Assistant Professor, University of Washington, Seattle, Washington

DENNIS J. MCTIGUE, DDS, MS
Professor, Division of Pediatric Dentistry and Community Oral Health, College of Dentistry, Ohio State University, Columbus, Ohio

GARY NELSON, DDS, MS
Private Practice, Paradise; Department of Pediatric Dentistry, University of Washington, Seattle, Washington

TRAVIS NELSON, DDS, MSD, MPH
Acting Assistant Professor, Department of Pediatric Dentistry, University of Washington, Seattle, Washington

MAN WAI NG, DDS, MPH
Dentist-in-Chief, Boston Children's Hospital, Assistant Professor of Developmental Biology (Pediatric Dentistry), Harvard School of Dental Medicine, Boston, Massachusetts

AVINA PARANJPE, BDS, MS, MSD, PhD
Department of Endodontics, School of Dentistry, University of Washington, Seattle, Washington

BARBARA SHELLER, DDS, MSD
Orthodontist and Pediatric Dentist, Affiliate Professor, Departments of Orthodontics and Pediatric Dentistry, Seattle Children's Hospital, School of Dentistry, University of Washington, Seattle, Washington

H. JUNG SONG, DDS, MSD
Private Periodontal Practice, Edmonds; Attending Periodontist, Seattle Children's Hospital, Seattle; Department of Pediatric Dentistry, Affiliate Instructor for the Center for Pediatric, University of Washington Dental School, Seattle, Washington

ELIZABETH VELAN, DMD, MSD
Pediatric Dentist, Affiliate Assistant Professor, Department of Pediatric Dentistry, Seattle Children's Hospital, School of Dentistry, University of Washington, Seattle, Washington

Contents

> Early childhood caries (ECC), common in preschoolers, can lead to pain and infection if left untreated. Yet, ECC is largely preventable, and if it is identified early and the responsible risk factors are addressed, its progression can be halted or slowed. This article reviews the rationale for a first dental visit by age 1 year, caries risk assessment, and risk-based prevention and management of ECC and discusses strategies for providers to implement these contemporary evidence-based concepts into clinical practice.

> This article reviews periodontal disease and gingival disease and also explores issues relating to mucogingival defects such as gingival hyperplasia, gingival recession, and exposure of impacted canines.

> This overview covers diagnosis and management of the most common dental injuries in children and identifies those children at greatest risk. Crown fractures and luxation injuries in both the primary and permanent dentition are discussed and treatment options based on current international guidelines are detailed.

> Vital pulp therapy is performed to preserve the health status of the tooth and its ultimate position in the arch. These procedures are performed routinely in primary and permanent teeth. This review is divided into 2 parts: the first aims to illustrate the basic biology of the pulp and the effects on the pulp due to various procedures; the second focuses on the clinical aspects of treatment and the use of various dental materials during different vital pulp therapy procedures performed in the primary and permanent teeth.

> This article discusses contemporary pediatric restorative dentistry. Indications and contraindications for the choice of different restorative materials in different clinical situations, including the risk assessment of the patient,

are presented. The specific use of glass ionomer cement or resin-modified glass ionomer cement, resin-based composite, and stainless steel crowns is discussed so that preparation design and restoration placement is understood.

Pediatric Oral and Maxillofacial Surgery

Elizabeth Kutcipal

Pediatric oral and maxillofacial surgery is rarely seen as a separate entity from adult oral and maxillofacial surgery. Many procedures are similar on adults and children; however, children have unique behavioral, anatomic, and physiologic considerations. Children also have a propensity for certain injuries and pathologic lesions. Children born with congenital anomalies may also have a special subset of needs. This article is a brief review of oral and maxillofacial surgery on the pediatric population.

Temporomandibular Joint Disorders in Children

James A. Howard

A child's difficulty in verbalizing the precise location and nature of facial pain and jaw dysfunction often results in a nondefinitive history, increasing the importance of the dentist's awareness of the early signs and symptoms of temporomandibular joint disorders (TMD). A focused examination of the masticatory musculature, the temporomandibular joints, and associated capsular and ligamentous structures can reveal if a patient's symptoms are TMD in origin. An accurate differential diagnosis enables timely referral to appropriate health care providers and minimizes the use of diagnostic imaging.

The Continuum of Behavior Guidance

Travis Nelson

Behavior guidance is a continuum of techniques, basic and advanced, fundamental to the provision of quality dental care for pediatric patients. This practice must be individualized, pairing the correct method of behavior guidance with each child. To select the appropriate technique, the clinician must have a thorough understanding of each aspect of the continuum and anticipate parental expectations, child temperament, and the technical procedures necessary to complete care. By effectively using techniques within the continuum of behavior guidance, a healing relationship with the family is maintained while addressing dental disease and empowering the child to receive dental treatment throughout their lifetime.

The Role of Sedation in Contemporary Pediatric Dentistry

Travis Nelson and Gary Nelson

Procedural sedation offers an effective and humane way to deliver dental care to the young, anxious child and to those with extensive treatment needs. Delivery of sedation requires thorough understanding of its indications and contraindications, patient assessment, pharmacology, monitoring, and office protocol. Safe and successful outcomes depend on a systematic approach to care, and the ability to manage unintended cardiopulmonary events.

This article discusses aspects of providing dental treatment in hospitals to patients with complex medical and/or behavioral problems. Practical information for patient selection for care in a hospital operating room, obtaining hospital privileges, and other aspects of dental care in hospitals are introduced.

DENTAL CLINICS OF NORTH AMERICA

DOWNLOAD Free App!

Review Articles
THE CLINICS

NOW AVAILABLE FOR YOUR iPhone and iPad

Preface

Pediatric Dentistry

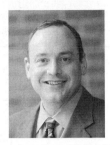

Joel H. Berg, DDS, MS
Guest Editor

This special issue provides information to those managing the oral health of children. In addition to the usual subjects presented in other publications, such as caries, prevention and restorative dentistry, as well as behavior management, we have added some special articles on oral surgery, temporomandibular disorders, and periodontal issues, all focused on children. It is hoped that this comprehensive review of clinical oral care for children will provide important information that will improve the care of all children.

WHAT IS PEDIATRIC DENTISTRY?

Pediatric dentistry is an age-defined specialty that provides both primary and comprehensive preventive and therapeutic oral health care for infants and children through adolescence, including those with special health care needs.[1] It is one of the 9 recognized dental specialties of the American Dental Association. Pediatric dentists complete 2 to 3 years of additional specialized training (after the required 4 years of dental school) to prepare them for treating a wide variety of children's dental problems.[2]

Pediatric dental practitioners represent approximately 8400 professionals in the United States who specialize in pediatric oral health care and serve as primary care and specialty providers for millions of children and youth.

They also serve as the primary contributors to education programs and scholarly works concerning children's dental care. And, pediatric dentistry encompasses general dentists who treat a significant number of children in their practices.

PEDIATRIC DENTISTRY ORAL HEALTH POLICIES AND CLINICAL GUIDELINES

The national academy—with which pediatric dentists align to remain current on practice issues, new products, technologies, and pediatric dental guidelines and policy updates—is the American Academy of Pediatric Dentistry (AAPD). The AAPD sets the standard for pediatric oral health care in terms of authoritative development and the publishing of pediatric oral health policies, clinical guidelines, and public advocacy.

Dent Clin N Am 57 (2013) ix–xiv
http://dx.doi.org/10.1016/j.cden.2012.10.002
0011-8532/13/$ – see front matter © 2013 Elsevier Inc. All rights reserved.

These include advocacy for children's oral health care before legislative and government agencies, dissemination of information to parents, guardians, and other caregivers about children's oral health care, and continuing professional education for pediatric dentists and general dentists who treat children. The AAPD's top organizational priority is to secure financial access to quality oral health care for all children, pursuing this agenda at the national and state level. [3]

Although AAPD guidelines and policies serve as the backbone for the quality of care we deliver, in the most practical sense, those of us who train and practice as pediatric dentists do so because we take to heart the impact we can make in children's overall health, well-being, and quality of life.

Practically speaking, we serve children and families by providing medically necessary care; we educate and influence positive oral health behavior and fluoride use and do everything we can to help reverse the growing trend—now at epidemic levels—of early childhood caries (ECC) disease in the United States.[4]

Medically Necessary Care

Medically Necessary Care (MNC) is the reasonable and essential diagnostic, preventive, and treatment services, including supplies, appliances, and devices, and follow-up care as determined by qualified health care providers in treating any condition, disease, injury, or congenital or developmental malformation. MNC includes all supportive health care services that, in the judgment of the attending dentist, are necessary for the provision of optimal quality therapeutic and preventive oral care. These services include, but are not limited to, sedation, general anesthesia, and utilization of surgical facilities. MNC always takes into account the patient's age, developmental status, and psychosocial well-being in addition to the setting appropriate to meet the needs of the patient and family.[5]

The Practice and Prevention of Early Childhood Caries Disease

Childhood caries as a common chronic disease results from an imbalance of multiple risk factors and protective factors over time. To decrease the risk of developing ECC, professional and at-home preventive measures are important. These include decreasing the parent's/siblings' transmission of the cariogenic bacteria that causes cavities, minimizing saliva-sharing activities, and implementing oral hygiene measures no later than the time of eruption of the first primary tooth.[6]

Furthermore, tooth brushing should be performed for children by a parent twice daily, using a soft toothbrush of age-appropriate size. In children considered at moderate or high risk for caries under the age of 2, a "smear" of fluoridated toothpaste should be used. In all children ages 2 to 5, a "pea-size" amount should be used.[6]

In additional, it is recommended that families establish a dental home within 6 months of the eruption of the first tooth and no later than 12 months of age. This timing is critical in order to conduct a caries risk assessment and to provide parental education including anticipatory guidance for prevention of oral diseases. Guidance at this point typically covers the importance of avoiding the high-frequency consumption of liquids and/or solid foods containing sugar, especially sugar-containing beverages in a baby bottle or no-spill training cup. Finally, pediatric dental professionals will often work in concert with medical providers to ensure all infants and toddlers have access to dental screenings, counseling, and preventive procedures.[6]

EARLY CHILDHOOD CARIES DISEASE—RISK AND INTERVENTION

Today, a growing number of medical, dental, and political stakeholders have a vested interest in the topic of early caries risk assessment—because of its impact on the youngest members of our society. Never have we had greater access to risk assessment tools and methods for detecting and preventing dental caries in very young children. And yet, tooth decay affects children in the United States more than any other chronic infectious disease. The overall health impact of this disease in young children can be devastating. Untreated tooth decay causes pain and infections that may lead to problems with eating, speaking, playing, and learning.[4]

Children most at risk for developing ECC disease include those on Medicaid; children whose mother, siblings, or primary caregiver has cavities; children who are premature, low birth weight, or diabetic, or have other special health needs; and children who use a bottle after 15 months of age or have sweets and starchy snacks more than 3 times a day.[7]

Also of note is the need for an entirely different approach to intervention. Early intervention is about managing the disease well before it manifests as a cavity—since this is what typically initiates a toddler visit to the dentist. Early intervention also elevates the theme of education to include the family, related caregivers, and the community of health care providers—all of whom must be educated in the detection and prevention of ECC.

Inherent in this revolutionary approach is the prevailing theme of education: including the family and all related caregivers to the community of health care providers, all of whom need to be educated in the prevention of early childhood caries. An increased awareness of the detrimental effects of early childhood caries disease has prompted the involvement of key health care and policy stakeholders to address this pressing issue. Early childhood caries disease is behavioral; it is societal—in that we pay the costs for infant and toddler caries disease that goes unchecked—and it is preventable.[4] The potential for changing behavioral attitudes starts with the opportunity for early caries risk assessment—by age 1, along with the establishment of a dental home.[8] This represents one of the most effective and proactive ways to involve and educate parents. As well, medical and dental clinicians, working in concert, can ensure that the highest risk infants and toddlers are seen and treated.

As advocates of oral health, the AAPD, American Academy of Pediatrics, and the American Dental Association have a standing policy for children to have a dental home by age 1 (American Academy of Pediatrics 2003; American Academy of Pediatric Dentistry 2006). The recognition of the disease has led to a paradigm shift in prevention strategies and the implementation of policies for early examination.

EARLY CHILDHOOD CARIES DISEASE—MANAGEMENT AND THE CHALLENGES AHEAD
A New Paradigm: The Total Health Team

There is a growing awareness of the importance of oral health among non-dental health professionals, due in part to the Surgeon General's Report on Oral Health.[9] This report highlighted the substantial national burden from oral diseases and the existence of oral health disparities in vulnerable populations. The release of the report, *The Face of the Child: Surgeon General's Conference on Children and Oral Health,* further considered issues of relevance to pediatric oral health.[10]

The American Academy of Pediatrics states that the first oral health screening should take place at or around 6 months, likely in conjunction with a checkup already on the docket as part of the routine schedule of well-baby examinations.[8] Although integrating an oral assessment into an existing well-baby examination sounds like the right thing to do, this approach has never gained traction. And, as with any "system" of health care delivery, access to the most appropriate care for all must target those at greatest risk as early as possible in the course of potential disease. Furthermore, there must be a mechanism in place to provide continuous, comprehensive, and effective preventive and surgical care where it is needed most. This would focus the attention and resources on those infants and toddlers deemed at greatest risk. To that end, it is imperative for dental, medical, and other health professionals to work together effectively—across their practices and in their communities—to promote the oral health of children.

ECC: An Infectious Disease and Third Party Call-to-Action

For the prevalence of dental caries to be reduced, the disease must be viewed as an infectious disease. As with all infectious diseases, prevention is paramount in controlling the initiation and progression of the disease.[11]

It must also be noted that third-party payers hold an enormous amount of influence over the determination of who gets care when and how often. Third-party payers are recognizing the problem of waiting until children are older before providing for intervention.

As well, legislators are learning about the importance of early oral health. It is likely that as funding priorities are adjusted going forward, an increased awareness about the importance of early childhood intervention to achieve oral health in all children will help direct more financial investment in the management of dental caries prevention.

Parents are engaged early on help simply by virtue of their role, but clinicians are not talking with them enough—and at every possible opportunity—about their critical role in preventing and managing ECC in their infant or toddler.

Now is a very good time for every stakeholder who cares about early childhood oral health to ask the questions they need to ask. Stakeholders, by definition, have a vested interest in the well-being of the young children under their care. Given that position of caring, and with the multitude of touch points collectively managed by the various stakeholders, we have both the opportunity and the obligation to educate each stakeholder individually about their component role in managing children's oral health and preventing ECC.

FUTURE CONSIDERATIONS

Even though our knowledge of the biology of caries has contributed to enormous improvements in the prevalence of caries among adults and children in the United States, much of the trend toward improvements is attributed to fluoride in drinking water, dentifrice, and improved oral hygiene and dietary habits. And yet, in the past 10 years, we are seeing rapid declines in this positive trend for children.[4] Our knowledge of the disease process does not seem to be influencing significant enough reverse-trend changes in diet or behaviors.

A host of strategies has been proposed and implemented to address this pandemic, including screening and risk assessment by physicians and nurses, education by community partners, establishment of a dental home by 1 year of age, and media campaigns to inform and motivate positive and healthy dental habits by families.[12] This progress is counterbalanced by failures, unfortunately, and for those children most at-risk, future efforts and considerations must focus on answering some as-yet-unanswered questions, including the following:

- Why do some children in a family get cavities, while others who have the same diet and hygiene habits do not?
- Are *Mutans streptococci* really the main acidogenic bacteria responsible for caries or are there other bacteria that are not as easily cultivable?

- What new tools and techniques can we use to detect caries risk prior to the development of the disease?
- When children at risk for caries are identified early, what can be done to truly prevent the disease from occurring?
- Once the disease process has begun, what is the best way to manage the disease and to minimize the consequences of the disease?

These important questions fall into 4 categories: identifying new cariogenic micro-flora, host factors and caries susceptibility, caries-risk prediction, and dental materials and disease management.[12] Prevention and management of this epidemic disease will be best accomplished by coordinating efforts with individuals and groups who are likewise dedicated to the well-being of children. Together, we can make a difference in the lives of these youngest citizens.

Joel H. Berg, DDS, MS
University of Washington School of Dentistry
HSB D-322, Box 356365
Seattle, WA 98195, USA

E-mail address:
joelberg@uw.edu

REFERENCES

1. American Dental Association Commission on Dental Accreditation. Accreditation standards for advanced specialty education programs in pediatric dentistry. Commission on Dental Accreditation, Chicago: 2000.
2. American Academy of Pediatric Dentistry (AAPD). President's Message. Available at: http://www.aapd.org/about/. Accessed May, 2012.
3. American Academy of Pediatric Dentistry Core Values. Revised 2009. Available at: http://www.aapd.org/media/Policies_Guidelines/CoreValues.pdf. Accessed September, 2009.
4. Department of Health and Human Services, Centers for Disease Control and Prevention, Children's Oral Health [Homepage on the internet], [Updated January 7, 2011]. Available at: http://www.cdc.gov/OralHealth/topics/child.htm. Accessed January 7, 2011.
5. American Academy of Pediatric Dentistry. Definition of Medically Necessary Care. Revised 2011. Available at: http://www.aapd.org/media/Policies_Guidelines/D_MedicallyNecessaryCare.pdf. Accessed September, 2011.
6. American Academy of Pediatric Dentistry. Policy on Early Childhood Caries (ECC): Classifications, Consequences, and Preventive Strategies. Revised 2011. Available at: http://www.aapd.org/media/Policies_Guidelines/P_ECCClassifications.pdf.
7. Dye BA, Tan S, Smith V, et al. Trends in oral health status; United States, 1988-1994 and 1999-2004. National Center for Health Statistics. Vital Health Stat 2007;11(248):248–51.
8. American Academy of Pediatrics. Policy statement: Oral health risk assessment timing and establishment of the dental home. Pediatrics 2003;111:1110–3.
9. U.S. Department of Health and Human Services. Oral Health in America: A Report of the Surgeon General-Executive Summary. http://www.nidcr.nih.gov/AboutNIDCR/SurgeonGeneral/default.htm. Accessed October, 2000. Rockville (MD): U.S. Department of Health and Human Services, National Institute of Dental and Craniofacial Research, National Institutes of Health; 2000.

10. Surgeon General's Conference on Children and Oral Health, June 11-12, 2000. Washington, DC: http://www/nidcr.nih.gov/AboutNIDCR/SurgeonGeneral/Children.htm. Accessed October, 2000.
11. Donly K. Managing caries: Obtaining arrest. In: Berg JH, Slayton RL, editors. Early childhood oral health. Ames (IA): Wiley-Blackwell; 2009.
12. Slayton R. Future directions. In: Berg JH, Slayton RL, editors. Early childhood oral health. Ames (IA): Wiley-Blackwell; 2009.

Early Childhood Caries
Risk-Based Disease Prevention and Management

Man Wai Ng, DDS, MPH[a,b,*], Isabelle Chase, DDS[a,b]

KEYWORDS

- Early childhood caries • Caries risk assessment • Risk-based disease
- Prevention and management

KEY POINTS

- Early childhood caries (ECC), a common chronic disease that can progress rapidly if left untreated, is largely preventable.
- To reduce the risk of ECC, children should have a first dental visit and establish a dental home by 1 year of age to receive risk-based primary prevention and counseling.
- ECC cannot be addressed successfully by restorative treatment alone and requires changes to dietary and oral hygiene practices.
- If ECC is identified early and the responsible risk factors are addressed, the progression of ECC can be halted or slowed.
- Effective ECC management requires using risk-based disease prevention and management approaches that include caries risk assessment, self-management goals, and caries remineralization strategies.

INTRODUCTION

Early childhood caries (ECC) is the most common chronic condition among children in the United States. In 2-year-olds to 5-year-olds, caries rates are on the increase, having increased 15% in recent years to 28%.[1] Children of minority or low-income families are disproportionately affected[2,3] and are less likely to receive timely care.[3,4]

ECC is a particularly virulent form of caries that affects the primary teeth of infants and preschool children. Typically, decay begins on the maxillary incisors followed by maxillary and mandibular molars, affecting teeth sequentially as they erupt. ECC can progress rapidly if left untreated, resulting in pain and infection. Yet, ECC is largely

Funding Sources: Dr Ng: DentaQuest Institute and DentaQuest Foundation supported grants. Dr Chase: None.
Conflict of Interest: Dr Ng: Steering committee member of DentaQuest Institute supported National Oral Health Quality Improvement Committee. Dr Chase: None.
[a] Boston Children's Hospital, 300 Longwood Avenue, Boston, MA 02115, USA; [b] Harvard School of Dental Medicine, 188 Longwood Avenue, Boston, MA 02115, USA
* Corresponding author. Boston Children's Hospital, 300 Longwood Avenue, Boston, MA 02115.
E-mail address: Manwai.ng@childrens.harvard.edu

preventable,[5,6] and if it is identified early and the responsible risk factors are addressed, its progression can be halted or slowed.[6,7]

ECC: CAUSE

Dental caries is a multifactorial disease caused by oral bacteria and mediated by dietary sugars and carbohydrates. It is well established that caries is a dynamic process that can progress or regress, depending on a multitude of variables that can alter the normal balance of demineralization and remineralization.[8,9] The Featherstone caries balance concept[8] states that the balance of pathologic factors can be altered in favor of protective factors to halt or slow down the caries process. In individuals with active caries, without changes to alter the balance in favor of protective factors over pathologic factors, the caries process continues, with new and recurrent caries resulting.

The mutans streptococci (MS) group of bacteria is most strongly associated with the pathogenic process of ECC.[10–13] MS adheres to enamel and produces large amounts of acids but it also thrives in the acidic environment it creates. MS can be acquired during early infancy through vertical transmission of bacteria via saliva from the primary adult caregiver to the child.[14] Factors influencing colonization include frequent sugar exposure in infants and habits that allow salivary transfer from mothers to their infants. Maternal factors that increase bacterial transmission to their infants include high levels of MS, poor plaque control, and frequent intake of sugars and carbohydrates.[13]

Children's risk for caries development and progression is influenced by various social and behavioral factors,[15] including diet, oral hygiene practices, and fluoride exposure.[16,17] Parents help define oral health practices early in their child's life and also when to establish regular dental care. Their beliefs and self-efficacy help determine to what extent they engage in oral health-promoting behaviors.[18,19]

INFANT ORAL HEALTH AND ESTABLISHMENT OF A DENTAL HOME

The American Dental Association (ADA),[20] American Academy of Pediatric Dentistry (AAPD),[21] and American Academy of Pediatrics[22] recommend that all children have their first preventive dental visit and establishment of a dental home by age 1 year. A dental home is defined as an ongoing, comprehensive relationship between the dentist and the patient (and parents), inclusive of all aspects of oral health delivered in a continuously accessible, coordinated, and family-centered way.[23] A dental home should be established such that children can have access to regular dental visits that include caries risk assessment (CRA), anticipatory guidance, and individualized plans to prevent and manage disease, with referral to dental specialists when appropriate.

Preventing ECC is more cost-effective compared with treating advanced caries.[24] An infant oral health visit and establishment of a dental home by age 1 year offer the best opportunity to provide risk-based primary prevention and promote sound oral health practices, which can mitigate a child's risk of disease over a lifetime.

CRA

An assessment of caries risk during infancy and periodically thereafter allows for early identification and understanding of a child's current and changing risk factors for ECC. Previous experience of caries is a strong predictor of future caries.[25–27] Therefore, successfully addressing caries risk factors during early childhood can reduce a lifetime burden of dental disease.

Caries risk factors unique to infants and young children include perinatal considerations, establishment of oral flora and host-defense mechanisms, susceptibility of newly erupted teeth, dietary transition from bottle or breastfeeding to cups, and child-hood food preferences.[22] CRA allows for a customized preventive plan to be developed that is appropriate for the child and family.

Fig. 1 shows a CRA form adapted from the American Academy of Pediatric Dentistry (AAPD) CRA Form for 0-year-old to 5-year-old children.[27] **Fig. 2** shows a CRA tool used by in the ECC Collaborative,[28] a quality improvement initiative funded by the DentaQuest Institute, which is testing the feasibility and effectiveness of a risk-based disease management approach in preschool children with ECC. The ECC Collaborative CRA is an adaptation of the AAPD and pediatric Caries Management by Risk Assessment (CAMBRA) CRA.[6] The progression or reversal of dental caries is determined by the balance between pathologic and protective factors.

Biological risk factors are determined from an interview with the parent and include biological or lifestyle factors that contribute to the development or progression of caries. These factors include a mother with active decay or recently placed restorations, a family of low economic status, a child who frequently consumes snacks and drinks that are high in sugars or carbohydrates, and a child who sleeps with a bottle or sippy cup containing anything other than water. Children with special health care needs (SHCN) may have feeding problems as well as difficulties with food clearance.

Protective factors, also determined during the interview with the parent, include biological or behavioral factors that can improve a child's caries risk. These factors include assistance with toothbrushing and optimal exposure to fluoride.

Disease indicators are clinical findings from the examination that correlate strongly to disease or to improved caries risk. These indicators include the presence of cavitated lesions, enamel demineralization, enamel defects, presence of heavy plaque (leading to gingival inflammation), and remineralization. Children born prematurely, or with low birth weight, or those with SHCN are at increased risk for enamel defects. Teeth with enamel defects in the presence of poor plaque control and frequent sugar or carbohydrate exposure are at significant risk for ECC.

Based on the distribution of risk factors and protective factors, the health care provider can make a determination of a child's caries risk, explain the caries process and the causative factors to the parent, and develop in collaboration with the parent self-management goals to prevent or manage their child's caries risk.

ECC DISEASE PREVENTION AND MANAGEMENT STRATEGIES

Children's oral health is influenced by various social and behavioral factors, such as diet, oral hygiene practices, and fluoride exposure. It is now accepted that surgical treatment of caries alone does not address the caries process.[9] On the other hand, it is known that caries is preventable and the disease may be halted or slowed down under a favorable balance of conditions. Therefore, risk-based disease management of ECC is based on the assumption that children who initially present as high caries risk may improve their caries risk over time.

Delaying the Transmission of Oral Bacteria in Infants

Preventing and delaying the acquisition and transmission of MS involve reducing the bacteria levels in the mother and other caregivers, modifying saliva-sharing activities, and altering feeding behaviors that promote caries.[21] Mothers and adult caregivers should be encouraged to seek dental care and improve their own oral health, ideally in the prenatal period.[21]

	High Risk	Moderate Risk	Protective
Risk (Biological) Factors			
Mother/primary caregiver has active cavities	Yes		
Parent/caregiver has low socioeconomic status	Yes		
Child has >3 between meal sugar-containing snacks or beverages per day	Yes		
Child is put to bed with bottle containing natural or added sugar	Yes		
Child has special health care needs		Yes	
Child is a recent immigrant		Yes	
Protective Factors			
Child receives optimally fluoridated drinking water or fluoride supplements			Yes
Child has teeth brushed daily with fluoridated toothpaste			Yes
Child receives topical fluoride from health professional			Yes
Child has dental home/regular dental care			Yes
Clinical Findings (Disease Indicators)			
Child has > 1 decayed/missing/filled surfaces	Yes		
Child has white spot lesions or enamel defects	Yes		
Child has elevated mutans streptococci levels	Yes		
Child has plaque on teeth		Yes	

Fig. 1. CRA form for 0-year-olds to 5-year-olds. (*Adapted from* American Academy of Pediatric Dentistry (AAPD). Guideline on caries-risk assessment and management for infants, children and adolescents. Chicago (IL): American Academy of Pediatric Dentistry (AAPD); 2011; with permission.)

Patient's First Name	Last Name	MRN	Name of Provider	Today's Date / /
				Child's DOB / /

Type of visit: (Circle all that apply)

Initial	Recall	DM	Fluoride Varnish	Restorative	ITR	Sealants	Sedation	Emergency	OR	Other

CAN BE COMPLETED BY CLINICAL STAFF, PATIENT OR DENTIST

Biologic Factors | | *Comments*
Child has history of active caries	Y N	
Mother has active caries	Y N	
Siblings have active caries	Y N	
Continuous bottle use	Y N SW	
Sleeps with bottle or nurses on demand	Y N SW	Describe
Juice/milk in Sippy cup	Y N SW	Describe
Frequent snacking	Y N SW	Describe
SHCN	Y N	
Potential caries causing medications	Y N	Describe

Protective Factors

Tooth brushing	Y N	__x/day
Assistance with brushing	Y N SW	
Fluoride toothpaste	Y N	__x/day
Topical fluoride (Gelkam, Prevident, ACT)	Y N	__x/day
Floss	Y N NA	
Drinks fluoridated water	Y N	

TO BE COMPLETED BY DENTIST

Disease Indicators/Risk Factors (from Clinical Examination)

Cavitation	Y N	Where
New Cavitation	Y N NA	
Demineralization / New Demin (WS)	Y N	Where
Radiographic decay	Y N NA	Where
Enamel defects	Y N	Where
Visible plaque	Y N SW	Where
Gingivitis	Y N Improved	Describe
Deep pits/fissures	Y N	Where

Indicators of Improved Caries Risk (from Clinical Examination)

Remineralization	Y N SW	Where
New remineralization	Y N	Where
Meeting self-management goals	Y N SW NA	
Stannous fluoride staining	Y N NA	

Other

Pain due to untreated caries	Y N	Where
Referral to OR/sedation	Y N	
Behavior (Frankl score)	1 2 3 4	

Overall Caries Risk: Low Medium High

NV: ___ months for DM/F varnish and _____

Self management goals
1)
2)
F-toothpaste ___x/day   Gelkam ___x/day

Fig. 2. CRA tool (0–5 years of age) used in the ECC Collaborative. ACT, 0.05% sodium fluoride rinse; DM/F varnish, disease management/fluoride varnish; Gelkam, 0.4% stannous fluoride toothpaste; ITR, interim therapeutic restoration; MRN, medical record number; N, no; NA, not applicable; OR, operating room; Prevident, 1.1% sodium fluoride toothpaste or gel; SHCN, special health care needs; SW, somewhat; WS, white spot; Y, yes. (*From* Ramos-Gomez FJ, Crall J, Gansky SA, et al. Caries risk assessment appropriate for the age 1 visit (infants and toddlers). J Calif Dent Assoc 2007;35(10):687–702; with permission.)

Diet and Nutrition Counseling

Dietary factors and food choices are determinants of dental caries and other chronic conditions.[29] Increased risk of caries is significantly associated with frequent and total consumption of simple sugars.[30] Parents should be counseled on the importance of reducing the frequency of exposure to sugars and refined carbohydrates in foods and drinks. Parents should be recommended to:

- Breastfeed their infants
- Avoid bottle or sippy cup to bed with anything other than water
- Limit sugary foods and drinks, including fruit juices, to mealtimes
- Encourage a balanced diet and healthy snacking, such as fruits and vegetables

Oral Hygiene, Use of Fluorides and Other Remineralizing Agents

Because the quality of tooth cleaning is important, young children require assistance with toothbrushing from an adult caregiver, beginning with the first erupted tooth. With correct positioning (such as using a knee-to-knee position with 2 adults or by having an adult approach from behind the child's head), and retraction of the lips and cheeks, it should take no more than 1 minute to brush a young child's teeth. Flossing is indicated if there are any contacts between teeth (typically after 3–4 years of age for posterior teeth).

Fluoride toothpaste is an effective, safe, and cost-effective prevention tool for children.[21,31] The current recommendation by the AAPD is that all children 2 to 5 years of age should use a pea-sized amount of fluoride toothpaste, whereas children younger than age 2 years determined to be medium or high caries risk should use a smear of fluoride toothpaste.[21] In children younger than 2 years, the concern is the risk of mild fluorosis. However, young children are largely at risk for fluorosis when allowed to eat or lick toothpaste.[31] Because ECC is preventable and can be devastating and costly to treat, CRA is most important during infancy and periodically thereafter to ensure that children who would benefit from fluoride toothpaste are recommended by their health professionals to use it.

Drinking fluoridated water is the most convenient and cost-effective way to provide optimal fluoride benefits.[32] In suboptimally fluoridated communities, a fluoride supplement may be prescribed to children with high caries risk as recommended by the ADA.[33]

Professional topical fluoride treatments should be based on CRA. The AAPD and the ADA recommend the following intervals to receive a full-mouth topical fluoride treatment (fluoride varnish):

- Every 3 to 6 months for high-risk children[34,35]
- A minimum of every 6 months for moderate-risk children[34,35]

Low-risk children may not receive additional benefit from topical fluoride treatments in addition to what they receive from fluoridated drinking water and toothpaste.[34] Children with severe ECC and who already have demineralized enamel or cavitated carious lesions may benefit from more frequent professional topical fluoride applications than every 3 months to assist in controlling the caries process.[7]

Other fluoride compounds such as silver diamine fluoride[36] and stannous fluoride[37] may be more effective than sodium fluoride for topical applications. Topical iodine[36] and emerging products such as casein phosphopeptide and calcium phosphate[38,39] products are available for use in addition to fluorides to assist in controlling and reversing the caries process.

Xylitol

Xylitol is a sugar substitute that is a part of the polyol family, which includes sorbitol, mannitol, and malitol. Xylitol reduces plaque formation and bacterial adherence and inhibits enamel demineralization and MS. Studies have found that xylitol can reduce MS in plaque and saliva and can reduce caries in young children and their mothers, along with decreasing the transmission of MS from mother to child.[36]

In adults, chewing 4 to 10 g of xylitol in chewing gum divided into 3 to 7 times per day is effective in suppressing the bacterial load.[36] Xylitol is now also available in syrups and lozenges.[40] A study found that xylitol syrup (8 g/d) reduced ECC by 50% to 70% in children 15 to 25 months of age.[41] Another study found that gum or lozenges taken by children at 5 g per day resulted in 35% to 60% reduction of caries, with no difference between the delivery methods.[42]

Sealants and Interim Therapeutic Restorations

Any tooth surface with deep pits or grooves benefits from treatment with a bonded or glass ionomer sealant. Typically, permanent molars are candidates for sealants, but primary molars may also benefit from sealant placement, especially if caries has already developed on other primary molars with similar pit and fissure anatomy.[43]

If destruction of tooth structure by the caries process is minimal, arrest of the decay might be possible with remineralization of tooth structure.[36] Restorative treatment may be deferred if the disease can be stabilized.[44]

If decay has progressed mildly into dentin or caries arrest has not been achieved, interim therapeutic restorations (ITR) may be performed to achieve caries control.[6,43] The ITR procedure involves removal of caries using hand or slow-speed rotary instruments with caution not to expose the pulp. After preparation, the tooth is restored with a fluoride-releasing glass ionomer restorative material. Parents should be advised that this approach is caries control rather than permanent restoration.[43]

Restorative Treatment

When significant tooth structure has been destroyed by the caries process, restorative treatment is performed to restore function or to improve esthetics. Young children who are not cooperative or children with SHCN commonly require pharmacologic management, including the use of nitrous oxide, sedation, or general anesthesia. However, the costs of general anesthesia are high,[45–48] and rates of recurrent caries after restorative treatment under general anesthesia have been reported in the literature to be 37% to 79% 6 to 12 months after.[49–52] Therefore, long-term success of restorative treatment is contingent on effective management of the disease responsible for ECC, along with the use of appropriate restorative technique and restorative materials for the primary dentition.[9]

Reevaluation of a child's caries risk status and compliance with self-management goals provides important information to determine the type of restorations best suited for each patient. A child who shows improved caries risk may receive more conservative restorative treatment. On the other hand, a child showing no improvement of caries risk or worsening clinical caries activity benefits from more aggressive care to reduce caries in susceptible tooth surfaces, such as with stainless steel crowns.[43]

When there is caries arrest, restorative treatment may be deferred,[36] especially in a child unable to cooperate for restorative care.[7] However, close follow-up and preventive care based on caries risk are essential to safeguard from relapse. Seeing a child more frequently for preventive care over time usually reduces a child's fears and builds trust between the care provider and the child, allowing for restorative treatment to be completed with greater ease in the clinical setting, at a later time.

IMPLEMENTING RISK-BASED ECC DISEASE PREVENTION AND MANAGEMENT INTO PRACTICE

Contemporary approaches to caries prevention and management, modeled after medical management of chronic conditions, such as diabetes and asthma, have been published in the dental literature.[6,7,9] Chronic disease management differs from a traditional approach of telling patients what to do. Instead, patients are assumed to have a responsibility for their own health and to play a central role in determining the care of their chronic conditions. It requires an active, informed patient and collaboration between the health care provider and the patient, ideally in a culturally and linguistically appropriate manner. An informed patient assists in selecting self-management goals to improve their disease risk. Treatment decisions are based on evidence-based guidelines. Risk-based disease prevention and management of ECC requires family engagement in day-to-day behavior modifications (eg, toothbrushing, topical fluorides and dietary control) that address disease cause.[7]

A risk-based disease management approach to address preschool children with ECC has been successfully implemented in a demonstration project at 2 hospital-based dental practices and has shown better clinical outcomes than the conventional approach to caries management. Thirty months of results found that children in the disease management group experienced lower rates of new cavitated lesions, pain, and referrals for restorative treatment under general anesthesia in the operating room. At 1 site, the disease management group experienced a 62% lower risk of new cavitation compared with a historical control group with ECC.[7]

Interviews with parents found that most believed the disease management protocol to be helpful for their children. Almost all parents appreciated given reasons as to why their children may have developed ECC. Some liked the partnership relationships with providers and to be given a voice in the dental care of their children.[7] An ECC Collaborative is presently testing the feasibility and effectiveness of the disease prevention and management of ECC approach in 7 diverse dental care settings that care for children at high risk for caries.[28]

DISEASE MANAGEMENT OF ECC

The disease management approach is contingent on accepting that a patient's caries risk status is not static, but can change over time. CRA and self-management goals are the cornerstone of risk-based disease prevention and management of ECC.[9]

Clinical Examination and Charting of Caries

Fig. 3 presents the International Caries Detection and Assessment System (ICDAS)[53-55] along with 2 alternative systems based on the ICDAS used by dental practices in the ECC Collaborative. **Fig. 4** defines the codes used in the International ICDAS and in alternative caries charting systems and describes the characteristics of the carious lesions.[55] A clinical examination and charting by tooth and surface of caries presence and activity using the ICDAS or alternative systems provides information important for determining the preventive and restorative treatment plan appropriate for the patient. Caries activity is determined by using a balled explorer or by gently sliding a sharp explorer over exposed dentin.

During an initial examination, accurate clinical assessment may be hampered by the presence of heavy plaque and patient cooperation. A 1-month follow-up visit allows for a more accurate assessment of demineralized enamel, remineralized enamel, and pit and fissure caries. Caries may progress and arrest at the same time in different locations of the dentition.

←———— Clinical Visual Assessment ————→

ICDAS Dental Terms	ICDAS Detection	ICDAS Activity	Alternative Charting System 1		Alternative Charting System 2		
Extensive cavity with visible dentin	6	+/-	6	A, B, C	D2A	D2B	D2C
Distinct cavity with visible dentin	5	+/-	5	A, B, C	D2A	D2B	D2C
Underlying dentin shadow	4	+/-	4	--	D2	--	--
Localized enamel breakdown	3	+/-	3	--	D1.5	--	--
Distinct visual change in enamel	2	+/-	2	--	D1	--	--
First visual change in enamel	1	+/-	2	--	D1	--	--
Sound	0	+/-	0	--	--	--	--

Fig. 3. The ICDAS and alternative ICDAS-based caries charting systems. The codes D1, D1.5, and D2 describe enamel or dentin changes, breakdown or cavitation: D1, enamel change; D1.5, enamel breakdown; D2, caries extending into dentin. The codes A, B, and C describe caries activity: A, completely arrested (inactive caries; may appear shiny or dark brown/black; feels hard); B, becoming inactive (may feel leathery or harder); C, active caries (feels soft). (*Adapted from* ICDAS Foundation. International Caries Detection and Assessment System. What is ICDAS? Available at: http://www.icdas.org/what-is-icdas. Accessed August 26, 2012; with permission.)

ICDAS Code	Alternative Codes 1 or 2	Characteristics of Lesion	
		Active Lesion	**Inactive Lesion**
1,2 or 3	**2 or 3** **D1 or D1.5**	• Surface of enamel is whitish/yellowish opaque with loss of luster • Feels rough when tip of probe is moved gently across the surface. • Lesion is in a plaque stagnation area, i.e.: pits and fissures, near gingival and approximal surface below contact point	• Surface of enamel is whitish, brownish or black • Enamel may be shiny and feels hard and smooth when tip of probe is moved gently across surface. • For smooth surfaces, caries lesion is typically located at some distance from gingival margin
4	**4 or D2**	• Probably active	
5 or 6	**5A,B or C** **D2A, B or C**	• Cavity feels soft or leathery on gently probing the dentin	• Cavity may be shiny and feels hard on gently probing the dentin

Fig. 4. Definitions of the codes used in the ICDAS and alternative caries charting systems, and characteristics of the carious lesions. (*Adapted from* International Caries Detection and Assessment System (ICDAS) Coordinating Committee. Appendix: Criteria Manual International Caries Detection and Assessment System (ICDAS II). Baltimore, MD: ICDAS. Revised in December and July 2009; with permission.)

Self-Management Goals

Fig. 5 shows a self-management goals handout for caregivers from CAMBRA.[5] The pathologic factors identified from the CRA interview with the parent are presented as a menu of self-management goals for the caregiver to select from and to work on at home before the next visit.

Box 1 shows a patient example using self-management goals for a 2-year-old child at high risk for caries. In the ECC Collaborative, brushing or applying 0.4% stannous fluoride to cavitated carious lesions 2 or more times per day is recommended. Interested parents are also informed about xylitol and casein phosphate products.

Disease Management Protocol

Fig. 6 shows an example of a disease management protocol, used in the ECC Collaborative, with return visit intervals based on the most recent caries risk status, in conjunction with restorative care as needed and as desired by the parent and

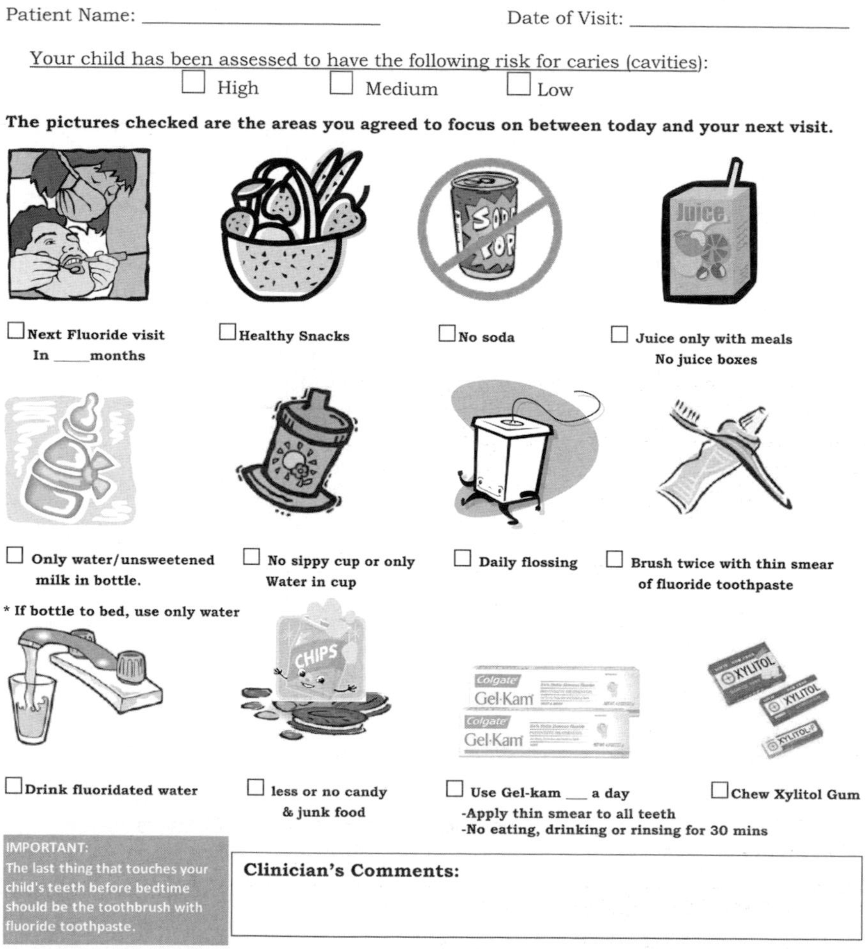

Patient Name: _____   Date of Visit: _____

Your child has been assessed to have the following risk for caries (cavities):

☐ High   ☐ Medium   ☐ Low

The pictures checked are the areas you agreed to focus on between today and your next visit.

☐ Next Fluoride visit In ____ months

☐ Healthy Snacks

☐ No soda

☐ Juice only with meals No juice boxes

☐ Only water/unsweetened milk in bottle.
* If bottle to bed, use only water

☐ No sippy cup or only Water in cup

☐ Daily flossing

☐ Brush twice with thin smear of fluoride toothpaste

☐ Drink fluoridated water

☐ less or no candy & junk food

☐ Use Gel-kam ___ a day
-Apply thin smear to all teeth
-No eating, drinking or rinsing for 30 mins

☐ Chew Xylitol Gum

IMPORTANT: The last thing that touches your child's teeth before bedtime should be the toothbrush with fluoride toothpaste.

Clinician's Comments:

Fig. 5. Self-management goals handout for caregivers. (*From* Ramos-Gomez FJ, Crall J, Gansky SA, et al. Caries risk assessment appropriate for the age 1 visit (infants and toddlers). J Calif Dent Assoc 2007;35(10):687–702; with permission.)

Box 1
Patient example

A 2-year-old child is deemed to be high caries risk because of the following contributing risk factors determined from a systematic CRA and clinical examination:

- Family history of caries
- Bottle to bed with milk
- Drinking juice in sippy cup throughout the day
- Frequent sugary and starchy snacks
- Brushing without adult assistance with fluoride-free training toothpaste
- Presence of heavy plaque, gingivitis, demineralized enamel, and mildly cavitated lesions

The parent would benefit from being given an explanation of the caries process and the causative factors to understand the conditions whereby the disease can progress or slow down (or even arrest). The parent should be asked if they are willing to partner with the care provider to control the disease process and to choose 2 self-management goals to work on until the next disease management visit.

The parent and dental provider may agree to these 2 self-management goals:

- Substituting water in bottle to bed
- Parent to assist child with fluoride toothpaste after breakfast and before bed

---

provider. In this protocol example, patients deemed to be high risk are recommended to return in 1 to 2 months, moderate-risk patients in 3 to 4 months, and low-risk patients in 6 to 12 months for reevaluation (with a new assessment of caries risk), fluoride varnish application, and ITR or restorative treatment as needed.

Box 2 shows an example of a disease management protocol for the 2-year-old child at high risk for caries. During each recall or subsequent disease management visit, a CRA is again performed, with a focus on inquiring about the risk factors specific to the child. Compliance or lack thereof with the agreed self-management goals is determined. A clinical examination is performed, reassessing for presence of new demineralization and cavitation along with caries remineralization. The findings are documented.

Practice Redesign to Support Disease Prevention and Management of Caries

For a successful paradigm shift to risk-based disease prevention and management to occur, a redesign of our care delivery systems is necessary. For example, care providers, patients, and families who are accustomed to the conventional surgical approach would have to be educated to accept an approach that emphasizes risk assessment, individualized disease prevention and management, and maintenance of health. Scheduling systems, which are typically set up to accommodate recall preventive visits every 6 months as allowed by insurance reimbursement, would have to be adjusted to allow more frequent preventive visits for patients at high risk for caries. Payment reform is also needed to reimburse providers for the time needed to perform CRA and provide teaching, education, and more frequent preventive care as needed based on the risk assessed.

Current models of oral health care delivery systems do not easily support risk-based disease prevention and management of caries. Quality improvement (QI) are concepts and methods used increasingly in health care to support redesign of care processes,

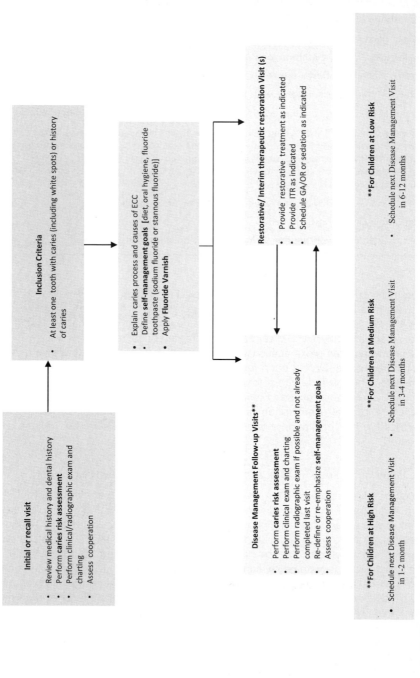

Initial or recall visit

- Review medical history and dental history
- Perform **caries risk assessment**
- Perform clinical/radiographic exam and charting
- Assess cooperation

Inclusion Criteria

- At least one tooth with caries (including white spots) or history of caries

- Explain caries process and causes of ECC
- Define **self-management goals** [diet, oral hygiene, fluoride toothpaste (sodium fluoride or stannous fluoride)]
- Apply **Fluoride Varnish**

Disease Management Follow-up Visits**

- Perform **caries risk assessment**
- Perform clinical exam and charting
- Perform radiographic exam if possible and not already completed last visit
- Re-define or re-emphasize **self-management goals**
- Assess cooperation

Restorative/ Interim therapeutic restoration Visit (s)

- Provide restorative treatment as indicated
- Provide ITR as indicated
- Schedule GA/OR or sedation as indicated

**For Children at High Risk

- Schedule next Disease Management Visit in 1-2 month

**For Children at Medium Risk

- Schedule next Disease Management Visit in 3-4 months

**For Children at Low Risk

- Schedule next Disease Management Visit in 6-12 months

Fig. 6. A disease management protocol (used in the ECC Collaborative). ECC, early childhood caries; GA/OR, general anesthesia/operating room; ITR, interim therapeutic restoration.

> **Box 2**
> **Patient example continues**
>
> The 2-year-old child at high risk for caries returns for a disease management follow-up visit in 1 month. There has been compliance with the agreed self-management goals. The clinical examination finds improved oral hygiene and some remineralization of the cavitated lesions. The child is still age-appropriately uncooperative. The parent is given positive reinforcement and agrees to limiting juice and snacking as a new self-management goal.
>
> After 1 or 2 additional 1-month disease management return visits, the patient is deemed medium risk and is recommended to return in 3 to 4 months for the next disease management visit and may receive ITR or conventional restorative care in the future, contingent on the clinical findings and the child's ability to cooperate in the clinical setting.
>
> On the other hand, if caries risk does not improve and the clinical caries worsens, sedation or general anesthesia can be considered and full-coverage restorations can be recommended.

based on a system of learning, incremental change, and incorporation of best practices from evaluating performance and outcomes.[56] QI methods, which use systematic data-guided activities, have helped sites in the ECC Collaborative to facilitate changes in their care delivery systems to support caries prevention and disease management in patient care. QI can be useful to guide improvements in many other oral care delivery systems and would accelerate the pace of adoption of innovative and evidence-based protocols into clinical practice.

SUMMARY

ECC cannot be successfully addressed by restorative treatment alone. A contemporary evidence-based clinical practice calls for early establishment of a dental home by age 1 year, use of CRA, self-management goals, and risk-based disease prevention and management of caries.

REFERENCES

1. Dye BA, Tan S, Smith V, et al. Trends in oral health status: United States, 1988-1994 and 1999-2004. Vital Health Stat 11 2007;(248):1–92.
2. Vargas CM, Ronzio CR. Disparities in early childhood caries. BMC Oral Health 2006;6(Suppl 1):S3.
3. Guarnizo-Herreno CC, Wehby GL. Explaining racial/ethnic disparities in children's dental health: a decomposition analysis. Am J Public Health 2012; 102(5):859–66.
4. Valencia A, Damiano P, Qian F, et al. Racial and ethnic disparities in utilization of dental services among children in Iowa: the Latino experience. Am J Public Health 2012. [Epub ahead of print].
5. Ramos-Gomez FJ, Crall J, Gansky SA, et al. Caries risk assessment appropriate for the age 1 visit (infants and toddlers). J Calif Dent Assoc 2007;35(10):687–702.
6. Ramos-Gomez F, Ng MW. Into the future: keeping healthy teeth caries free: pediatric CAMBRA protocols. J Calif Dent Assoc 2011;39(10):723–33.
7. Ng M, Torresyap G, White BA, et al. Disease management of early childhood caries: results of a pilot quality improvement project. J Health Care Poor Underserved 2012;23(Suppl 3):193–209.
8. Featherstone JD. Caries prevention and reversal based on the caries balance. Pediatr Dent 2006;28(2):128–32.

9. Fontana M, Wolff M. Translating the caries management paradigm into practice: challenges and opportunities. J Calif Dent Assoc 2011;39(10):702–8.
10. Loesche WJ. Role of *Streptococcus mutans* in human dental decay. Microbiol Rev 1986;50(4):353–80.
11. Berkowitz R. Etiology of nursing caries: a microbiologic perspective. J Public Health Dent 1996;56(1):51–4.
12. Ge Y, Caufield PW, Fisch GS, et al. *Streptococcus mutans* and *Streptococcus sanguinis* colonization correlated with caries experience in children. Caries Res 2008;42(6):444–8.
13. Berkowitz RJ. Causes, treatment and prevention of early childhood caries: a microbiologic perspective. J Can Dent Assoc 2003;69(5):304–7.
14. Berkowitz RJ. Mutans streptococci: acquisition and transmission. Pediatr Dent 2006;28(2):106–9 [discussion: 92–8].
15. Fisher-Owens SA, Gansky SA, Platt LJ, et al. Influences on children's oral health: a conceptual model. Pediatrics 2007;120(3):e510–20.
16. Yeung CA. Fluoride prevents caries among adults of all ages. Evid Based Dent 2007;8(3):72–3.
17. Weinstein P, Domoto P, Wohlers K, et al. Mexican-American parents with children at risk for baby bottle tooth decay: pilot study at a migrant farmworkers clinic. ASDC J Dent Child 1992;59(5):376–83.
18. Isong IA, Luff D, Perrin JM, et al. Parental perspectives of early childhood caries. Clin Pediatr (Phila) 2012;51(1):77–85.
19. Finlayson TL, Siefert K, Ismail AI, et al. Reliability and validity of brief measures of oral health-related knowledge, fatalism, and self-efficacy in mothers of African American children. Pediatr Dent 2005;27(5):422–8.
20. American Dental Association. Statement on early childhood caries. Available at: http://www.ada.org/2057.aspx. Accessed August 31, 2012.
21. American Academy of Pediatric Dentistry. Guideline on infant oral health care. Pediatr Dent 2011;33(6):124–8.
22. Preventive oral health intervention for pediatricians. Pediatrics 2008;122(6):1387–94.
23. Definition of dental home. Pediatr Dent 2011;33(6):12.
24. Lee JY, Bouwens TJ, Savage MF, et al. Examining the cost-effectiveness of early dental visits. Pediatr Dent 2006;28(2):102–5 [discussion: 92–8].
25. Bankel M, Robertson A, Kohler B. Carious lesions and caries risk predictors in a group of Swedish children 2 to 3 years of age. One year observation. Eur J Paediatr Dent 2011;12(4):215–9.
26. Fontana M, Santiago E, Eckert GJ, et al. Risk factors of caries progression in a Hispanic school-aged population. J Dent Res 2011;90(10):1189–96.
27. Guideline on caries-risk assessment and management for infants, children, and adolescents. Pediatr Dent 2011;33(6):110–7.
28. Early childhood caries phase 2 collaborative. Available at: http://www.dentaquestinstitute.org/improvement-initiatives/early-childhood-caries-initiative. Accessed August 26, 2012.
29. Cappelli DP, Mobley CC, editors. Prevention in clinical oral health. St Louis (MO): Mosby Elsevier; 2008.
30. Mobley C, Marshall TA, Milgrom P, et al. The contribution of dietary factors to dental caries and disparities in caries. Acad Pediatr 2009;9(6):410–4.
31. Do LG, Spencer AJ. Risk-benefit balance in the use of fluoride among young children. J Dent Res 2007;86(8):723–8.
32. CDC. Recommendations for using fluoride to prevent and control dental caries in the United States. MMWR Recomm Rep 2001;50(4414):1–42.

33. Rozier RG, Adair S, Graham F, et al. Evidence-based clinical recommendations on the prescription of dietary fluoride supplements for caries prevention: a report of the American Dental Association Council on Scientific Affairs. J Am Dent Assoc 2010;141(12):1480–9.

34. Professionally applied topical fluoride: evidence-based clinical recommendations. J Am Dent Assoc 2006;137(8):1151–9.

35. American Academy of Pediatric Dentistry. Guideline on fluoride therapy. Pediatr Dent 2011;33(6):153–6.

36. Milgrom P, Chi DL. Prevention-centered caries management strategies during critical periods in early childhood. J Calif Dent Assoc 2011;39(10):735–41.

37. Burke MR, Gambogi RJ, Simone AJ, et al. The scientific rationale and development of an optimized stannous fluoride dentifrice, Part 1. Compend Contin Educ Dent 1997;18(Spec No):2–9.

38. Turssi CP, Maeda FA, Messias DC, et al. Effect of potential remineralizing agents on acid softened enamel. Am J Dent 2011;24(3):165–8.

39. Robertson MA, Kau CH, English JD, et al. MI Paste Plus to prevent demineralization in orthodontic patients: a prospective randomized controlled trial. Am J Orthod Dentofacial Orthop 2011;140(5):660–8.

40. American Academy of Pediatric Dentistry. Guideline on xylitol use in caries prevention. Pediatr Dent 2011;33(6):157–60.

41. Milgrom P, Ly KA, Tut OK, et al. Xylitol pediatric topical oral syrup to prevent dental caries: a double-blind randomized clinical trial of efficacy. Arch Pediatr Adolesc Med 2009;163(7):601–7.

42. Alanen P, Isokangas P, Gutmann K. Xylitol candies in caries prevention: results of a field study in Estonian children. Community Dent Oral Epidemiol 2000;28(3):218–24.

43. American Academy of Pediatric Dentistry. Guideline on pediatric restorative dentistry. Pediatr Dent 2011;33(6):205–11.

44. Tinanoff N. Potential to improve oral health care through evidence, protocols, and payment models. J Public Health Dent 2012;72(Suppl 1):S48–51.

45. Duperon DF. Early childhood caries: a continuing dilemma. J Calif Dent Assoc 1995;23(2):15–6, 18, 20–2 passim.

46. Griffin SO, Gooch BF, Beltran E, et al. Dental services, costs, and factors associated with hospitalization for Medicaid-eligible children, Louisiana 1996-97. J Public Health Dent 2000;60(1):21–7.

47. Ramos-Gomez FJ, Huang GF, Masouredis CM, et al. Prevalence and treatment costs of infant caries in Northern California. ASDC J Dent Child 1996;63(2):108–12.

48. Kanellis MJ, Damiano PC, Momany ET. Medicaid costs associated with the hospitalization of young children for restorative dental treatment under general anesthesia. J Public Health Dent 2000;60(1):28–32.

49. Almeida AG, Roseman MM, Sheff M, et al. Future caries susceptibility in children with early childhood caries following treatment under general anesthesia. Pediatr Dent 2000;22(4):302–6.

50. Berkowitz RJ, Moss M, Billings RJ, et al. Clinical outcomes for nursing caries treated using general anesthesia. ASDC J Dent Child 1997;64(3):210–1, 228.

51. Eidelman E, Faibis S, Peretz B. A comparison of restorations for children with early childhood caries treated under general anesthesia or conscious sedation. Pediatr Dent 2000;22(1):33–7.

52. Graves CE, Berkowitz RJ, Proskin HM, et al. Clinical outcomes for early childhood caries: influence of aggressive dental surgery. J Dent Child (Chic) 2004;71(2):114–7.

53. Pitts N. "ICDAS"–an international system for caries detection and assessment being developed to facilitate caries epidemiology, research and appropriate clinical management. Community Dent Health 2004;21(3):193–8.

54. Ismail AI, Sohn W, Tellez M, et al. The International Caries Detection and Assessment System (ICDAS): an integrated system for measuring dental caries. Community Dent Oral Epidemiol 2007;35(3):170–8.

55. ICDAS Foundation. International Caries Detection and Assessment System. What is ICDAS? Available at: http://www.icdas.org/what-is-icdas. Accessed August 26, 2012.

56. Batalden PB, Davidoff F. What is "quality improvement" and how can it transform healthcare? Qual Saf Health Care 2007;16(1):2–3.

Periodontal Considerations for Children

H. Jung Song, DDS, MSD[a,b,c,*]

KEYWORDS

- Aggressive periodontitis • Gingival recession in children • Canine exposures
- Free gingival grafts • Implants in children • Gingival hyperplasia in children
- Drug-induced gingival overgrowth

KEY POINTS

- Maintenance and preservation of teeth and prevention of tooth loss are the main desired outcome of periodontal treatment.
- Minimal treatment for the maximum result outlines the main philosophy behind pediatric periodontics.
- A team approach must be considered for success in treating children.
- Close communication with pediatric dentists and other specialists, such as orthodontists, endodontists, and oral surgeons, are key to a successful outcome.

INTRODUCTION

Gingivitis and periodontitis are two different disease entities. Gingivitis is an inflammation of surrounding tissue without any bone loss, and periodontitis is inflammation with attachment loss. Typically, periodontitis is described as an irreversible process characterized by bone loss, while gingivitis is described as a reversible process limited to gingival tissue inflammation. The prevalence of periodontal disease in children and adolescents is relatively low, about 0.2% to 0.5%.[1] However, gingival disease and varying degrees of gingivitis are extremely common.[2]

Although nomenclature for gingival disease and mucogingival disease has stayed the same over time, periodontal disease in children has gone through many different

Disclosure: None.

Funding conflict: None.

[a] Private Periodontal Practice, Edmonds, WA, USA; [b] Department of Dentistry, Seattle Children's Hospital, 4800 Sand Point Way NE, Seattle, WA 98105, USA; [c] Department of Pediatrics, University of Washington Dental School, 1959 NE Pacific Street, Box 357136, Seattle, WA 98195, USA

* 21807 76th Avenue West, Edmonds WA 98026.

E-mail address: Jung@implants123.com

names over the last decade: periodontosis, prepubertal periodontitis, juvenile periodontitis and most currently aggressive periodontitis.

This article is divided into 2 subsets: periodontal disease and gingival disease, and mucogingival defects such as gingival hyperplasia, gingival recession, and exposure of impacted canines. Issues relating to trauma will also be visited briefly (**Box 1**).

PERIODONTITIS

Since 2009, periodontal disease in children and adolescents has been subcategorized into periodontitis as a manifestation of systemic disease, aggressive periodontitis, and necrotizing periodontal disease.[3] As with any disease, diagnosis and the defining of etiology are key to successful management of the patient's long-term periodontal health.

Periodontitis as a Manifestation of Systemic Disease

It is rare to see periodontitis as a manifestation of systemic disease in the general population. More commonly this disease entity is seen in hospital settings and special care settings. Examples of systemic diseases affecting periodontium include

Leukocyte adherence deficiency[4,5]
Congenital primary immunodeficiency[6]
Hypophosphatasia[7]
Chronic neutrophil defects[8,9]
Cyclic neutropenia[10]
Papillion Lefvre[11,12]
Down syndrome[13,14]

Diabetes is also considered to be a significant modifier of all forms of periodontal diseases. These affected individuals and their subgingival sites harbor *Actinobacillus actinomycetemcomitans* and *Capnocytophaga* Sp.[15]

Diagnostic criteria for periodontal disease as a manifestation of systemic disease includes[16]

Medical history, dental history, and appropriate radiographic evaluation
Full mouth probing and evaluation of presence of inflammation or infection
Identification of conditions suggestive of systemic disease, especially evaluation of the signs and symptoms
Request of laboratory test
Microbiological test
Consultation with primary or specialty care providers

The primary objective of periodontal care is to arrest infection and associated symptoms. Overall outcomes can be assessed by reduction of clinical signs of inflammation, reduction of probing depths, and control of acute symptoms (**Fig. 1**).[16]

Aggressive Periodontitis

When periodontitis appears in otherwise healthy patients with a rapid progression tendency, it can be categorized into aggressive periodontitis. Additionally, it can be subcategorized into localized or generalized depending on the degree of how many sites are affected within the individual (**Fig. 2**).

Diagnostic characteristics of localized aggressive periodontitis include

Circumpubertal onset
Periodontal damage being localized to permanent first molars and incisors

Box 1
Classification system for periodontal diseases and conditions

I. Gingival diseases

   A. Dental plaque-induced gingival diseases[a]

      1. Gingivitis associated with dental plaque only

         a. Without other local contributing factors

         b. With local contributing factors (see VIII.A)

      2. Gingival diseases modified by systemic factors

         a. Associated with the endocrine system

            1. Puberty-associated gingivitis

            2. Menstrual cycle-associated gingivitis

            3. Pregnancy-associated gingivitis and pyogenic granuloma

            4. Diabetes mellitus-assocated gingivitis

         b. Associated with blood dyscrasias

            1. Leukemia-associated gingivitis

            2. Other

      3. Gingival diseases modified by medications

         a. Drug-influenced gingival diseases

            1. Drug-influenced gingival enlargements

            2. Drug-influenced gingivitis

               a. Oral contraceptive-associated gingivitis

               b. Other

      4. Gingival diseases modified by malnutrition

         a. Ascorbic acid-deficiency gingivitis

         b. Other

   B. Nonplaque-induced gingival lesions

      1. Gingival diseases of specific bacterial origin

         a. *Neisseria gonorrhea*-associated lesions

         b. *Treponema pallidum*-associated lesions

         c. Streptococcal species-associated lesions

         d. Other

      2. Gingival diseases of viral origin

         a. Herpesvirus infections

            1. Primary herpetic gingivostomatitis

            2. Recurrent oral herpes

            3. Varicella zoster infections

         b. Other

      3. Gingival diseases of fungal origin

         a. *Candida* species infections

         b. Linear gingival erythema

      c. Histoplasmosis

      d. Other

    4. Gingival lesions of genetic origin

      a. Hereditary gingival fibromatosis

      b. Other

    5. Gingival manifestations of systemic conditions

      a. Mucocutaneous disorders

        1. Lichen planus

        2. Pemphigoid

        3. Pemphigus vulgaris

        4. Erythema multiforme

        5. Lupus erythematosus

        6. Drug-induced

        7. Other

      b. Allergic reactions

        1. Dental restorative materials

          a. Mercury

          b. Nickel

          c. Acrylic

          d. Other

        2. Reactions attributable to

          a. Toothpastes/dentifrices

          b. Mouth rinses/mouthwashes

          c. Chewing gum additives

          d. Foods and additives

        3. Other

    6. Traumatic lesions (factitious, iatrogenic, accidental)

      a. Chemical injury

      b. Physical injury

      c. Thermal injury

    7. Foreign body reactions

    8. Not otherwise specified

II. Chronic periodontitis[b]

  A. Localized

  B. Generalized

III. Aggressive periodontitis[b]

  A. Localized

  B. Generalized

IV. Periodontitis as a manifestation of systemic diseases

  A. Associated with hematological disorders

    1. Acquired neutropenia

    2. Leukemias

    3. Other

  B. Associated with genetic disorders

    1. Familial and cyclic neutropenia

    2. Down syndrome

    3. Leukocyte adhesion deficiency syndromes

    4. Papillon-Lefèvre syndrome

    5. Chediak-Higashi syndrome

    6. Histiocytosis syndromes

    7. Glycogen storage disease

    8. Infantile genetic agranulocytosis

    9. Cohen syndrome

    10. Ehlers-Danlos syndrome (types 4 and 8)

    11. Hypophosphatasia

    12. Other

  C. Not otherwise specified

V. Necrotizing periodontal diseases

  A. Necrotizing ulcerative gingivitis (NUG)

  B. Necrotizing ulcerative periodontitis (NUP)

VI. Abscesses of the periodontium

  A. Gingival abscess

  B. Periodontal abscess

  C. Pericoronal abscess

VII. Periodontitis associated with endodontic lesions

  A. Combined periodontic–endodontic lesions

VIII. Developmental or acquired deformities and conditions

  A. Localized tooth-related factors that modify or predispose to plaque-induced gingival diseases/periodontitis

    1. Tooth anatomic factors

    2. Dental restorations/appliances

    3. Root fractures

    4. Cervical root resorption and cemental tears

  B. Mucogingival deformities and conditions around teeth

    1. Gingival/soft tissue recession

     a. Facial or lingual surfaces

     b. Interproximal (papillary)

    2. Lack of keratinized gingiva

    3. Decreased vestibular depth

    4. Aberrant frenum/muscle position

5. Gingival excess

   a. Pseudopocket

   b. Inconsistent gingival margin

   c. Excessive gingival display

   d. Gingival enlargement (See I.A.3. and I.B.4.)

6. Abnormal color

C. Mucogingival deformities and conditions on edentulous ridges

   1. Vertical and/or horizontal ridge deficiency

   2. Lack of gingiva/keratinized tissue

   3. Gingival/soft tissue enlargement

   4. Aberrant frenum/muscle position

   5. Decreased vestibular depth

   6. Abnormal color

D. Occlusal trauma

   1. Primary occlusal trauma

   2. Secondary occlusal trauma

The periodontal conditions are categorized mainly into gingival diseases and periodontal diseases.

[a] Can occur on a periodontium with no attachment loss or on a periodontium with attachment loss that is not progressing.

[b] Can be further classified on the basis of extent and severity. As a general guide, extent can be characterized as Localized = ≤30% of sites involved and Generalized = >30% of sites involved. Severity can be characterized on the basis of the amount of clinical attachment loss (CAL) as follows: Slight = 1 or 2 mm CAL, Moderate = 3 or 4 mm CAL, and Severe = ≥5 mm CAL.

Reprinted from Armitage G. Development of a classification system for periodontal diseases and conditions. Ann Periodontol 1999;4:1–6; with permission from American Academy of Periodontology.

Microbiologic laboratory testing indicates *A actinomycetemcomitans*
Laboratory testing indicates neutrophil function abnormalities

Diagnostic characteristics for generalized aggressive periodontitis include[17]

Attachment loss of 4 mm or more affecting at least 8 teeth, at least 3 affected teeth other than molars and incisors
Patient is less than 35 years of age and has advanced attachment loss
Signs of early onset tooth loss
Most of the dentition, both primary and permanent, is affected
Inflammation of both marginal and attached gingiva

Treatment for aggressive periodontitis includes nonsurgical mechanical debridement such as scaling and root planning, control of local factors, occlusal therapy and periodontal surgery, as well as systemic antibiotics.[18]

The primary objective for periodontal treatment of localized and generalized aggressive periodontal disease includes elimination of microbial infection to halt disease progression. The main goal is to prevent tooth loss, maintenance of esthetics, and prevention of future attachment loss.[18]

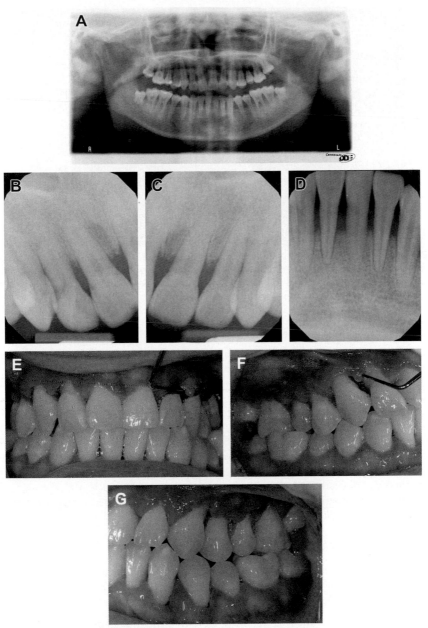

Fig. 1. (*A*) 18-year-old girl diagnosed with Crohn disease. Patient has recurrent periodontal abscess and is being treated both by surgical and nonsurgical means. (*B–D*) Crohn disease patient. Note the severe horizontal bone loss on the lower teeth. (*E–G*) Note severe inflammation and subgingival calculus.

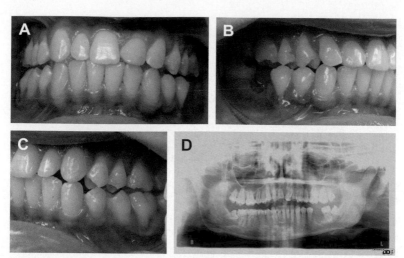

Fig. 2. (*A–D*) 17-year-old girld with Turner syndrome. Patient is deaf. Medications include levothyroxine, lisinopril, premarin, and vitamin D. A general dentist before the referral to periodontist recently extracted #19. Notice severe attachment loss. #9 is missing, and #11 is in the #9 position. #10 is transposed to the #11 position.

Necrotizing Periodontal Disease

Another category of periodontal disease seen in children and adolescents is necrotizing periodontal disease, formerly known as acute necrotizing ulcerative gingivitis (ANUG) or trench mouth.[3] This type of necrotizing periodontal disease is extremely rare in the general population of North America; however, developing countries in Africa, Asia, and South America show more frequent presentation, up to 2% to 5%.[19]

Offending microbiological and viral etiology includes *Provetella intermedia*, spirochetes, and viral infections such as human immunodeficiency syndrome (HIV), and herpesvirus.[20,21] Other confounding factors include lack of sleep, emotional stress, malnutrition, and a variety of systemic diseases.

Treatment includes mechanical debridement, oral hygiene instruction, and antibiotics such as metronidazole and penicillin (**Fig. 3**).[22]

MUCOGINGIVAL DISEASE

The American Academy of Periodontology defines mucogingival condition as a deviation from the normal anatomic relationship between the gingival margin and the mucogingival junction.[23] Most commonly seen mucogingival diseases in children include

Gingival recession relating to abnormal frenum attachment and decreased vestibular depths

Gingival hyperplasia such as gingival disease modified by medications and hereditary fibromatosis

Gingival issues associated with orthodontics including unerupted canines

Treatment modalities differ for each disease type, ranging from gingival augmentation therapy, root coverage, crown lengthening surgery, frenectomy, or exposure of unerupted teeth. However, the main objective for treatment outcome of the mucogingival disease is relatively the same. The desired outcome should result in correction of

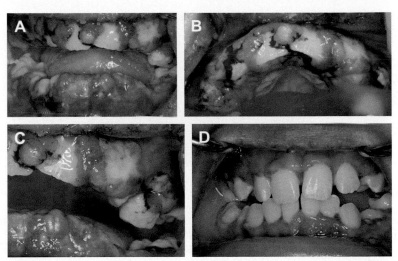

Fig. 3. (*A–C*) Gingival hyperplasia and heavy inflammation. It almost has the appearance of ANUG. (*D*) Postoperative pictures. Note significant improvements on the inflammation and gingival esthetics.

the mucogingival condition including lack of attached tissue, cessation of further recession, elimination of inflammation, and satisfactory esthetics.[23]

The unspoken rule of thumb for achieving an acceptable outcome is to improve the bad oral hygiene, since other etiologic factors such as genetics and certain medications are not elements within the clinician's control.

The following summarizes the gingival disease categories:

Gingival recession
Drug-induced gingival overgrowth (DIGO)
Gingival issues relating to orthodontics such as unerupted canines (labially positioned canines and palatally positioned canines) and localized juvenile spongiotic hyperplasia

Gingival Recession

When considering recession, one must be able to distinguish true recession from pseudorecession. True recession is an exposure of cementum with apical migration of the junctional epithelium.[24] The mandibular lower incisor region is most commonly seen often with abnormal frenum pull (**Figs. 4** and **5**).

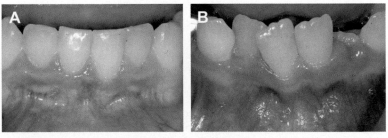

Fig. 4. Examples of pseudorecession. In (*A*), #24 has slightly more prominent root, and #23 is lingually placed. In (*B*), note the buccally rotated #25.

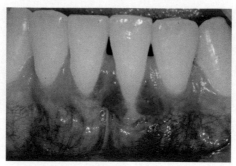

Fig. 5. Example of true recession. True recession is characterized by a lack of attached tissue and abnormal frenal attachment. Also note the highly inflamed tissue in the #24 site.

There is a long history of controversy surrounding when to correct these gingival recessions, and with regard to timing corrections with orthodontic therapies.[25–27] A close communication between the pediatric dentist, the orthodontist, and the periodontist is a crucial step in determining the prognosis of the receded teeth. Common sense can be a great tool too. If the receded tooth/teeth will be moved facially, resulting in stretching/thinning of gingiva, then mucoginigival surgery should be recommended before the orthodontic therapy. On the other hand, if orthodontics will move the affected tooth/teeth in a way to destretch the gingiva, then the mucogingival augmentation can wait until orthodontics has been completed.

A surgical treatment choice for lower anterior recession is a free gingival graft. Abnormal frenum attachment with shallow vestibule is a common etiology. However, frenectomy alone cannot improve the recession, hence frenectomy in conjunction with free gingival graft is indicated.[28] Despite the many different treatment choices such as connective tissue graft, lateral sliding graft, and coronally positioned graft for the mucogingival defect, due to the simplicity and speed of the surgery, an age-old, efficient, and effective free gingival technique is considered the treatment of choice most of the time.[29,30]

Although it is generally considered that root coverage is not possible, or extremely rare, with free gingival graft, the coverage depends on the details of the surgery such as incision and suturing design. Additionally, use of biologic materials such as Emdogain can improve the root coverage overall.

The treatment objectives for the recession via free gingival graft includes gaining attached tissue, elimination of frenum pull, deepening vestibule, and possible root coverage leading to eventual avoidance of tooth loss. Although Pasquinelli has reported new bone, cementum, and connective tissue attachment for human histologic studies after gingival graft surgery, it is generally accepted to have a long junctional epithelium attachment when root coverage happens with free gingival graft (**Figs. 6–9**).[31]

Drug-Induced Gingival Overgrowth

In contrast to recession, overgrowth of gingiva can be seen with or without any gingival inflammation. There are 2 main causes for the generalized gingival overgrowth, familiar and drug. It is commonly accepted that gingival overgrowth is dictated by genetic predilection with or without medication (**Fig. 10**).

Drugs associated with gingival enlargement can be broadly divided into 3 categories: anticonvulsants, calcium channel blockers, and immunosuppressants.

Not all patients placed on such drugs show gingival overgrowth. Most studies show that only a subset of patients treated with these medications will develop gingival

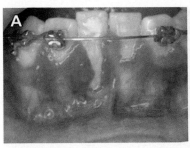
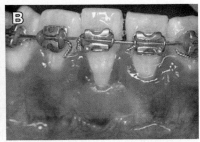

Fig. 6. Pre- and postsurgical pictures of most commonly seen gingival recession. Note the lack of attached tissue and shallow vestibule as well as abnormal frenum pulls on (*A*). Significant improvement on the attached tissue on (*B*).

overgrowth when oral hygiene is poor, hence when inflammation is vast. It is also suspected that there is a genetic predilection to gingival overgrowth (**Table 1**).

It is generally safe to assume that overgrown gingiva in phenytoin-treated patients is characterized by elevated levels of protein synthesis.[32] It is also reported that patients treated with cyclosporine A show reduced levels of matrix metalloproteinase MMP-1 and MMP-3 secretion, leading to increased accumulation of extracellular matrix components.[33]

Diagnosis of DIGO is mainly based on the clinical presentation and thorough history and examination. Most overgrowth starts at the papillary anterior facial gingiva areas, resulting in disfiguring esthetics and decreasing access for oral hygiene, leading to oral infection, caries, and acute periodontal abscess.

Due to esthetic considerations in the anterior region, it is important for both the patient and the patient's parents to understand the advantages of surgical treatment. Total or partial internal gingivectomy is suggested in literature.[34] Other treatment options include nonsurgical debridement,[35] uses of topical antifungal medications,[36,37] a short course of antibiotics (especially azithromycin),[38,39] carbon dioxide lasers,[40] and drug substitution and withdrawal.[36]

Because of the higher recurrence rate of gingival hyperplasia, some citing even up to 40% after treatment,[41] the patient and the patient's caregiver must be informed of potential additional surgical treatment in the future. To prevent recurrence, frequent maintenance visits and improved oral hygiene are recommended. An essix appliance

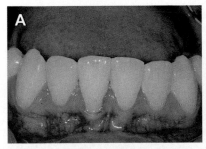
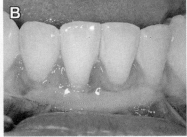

Fig. 7. (*A*) Before surgery. #25 has a slight recession and lack of attached tissue on both #24 and #25 sites with abnormal frenum pull. Note an extremely shallow vestibule. (*B*) After surgery. Significant improvements on the attached tissue level both #24 and #25 sites. Note a creeping attachment on the labial areas of #24.

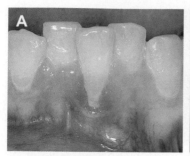 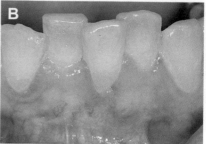

Fig. 8. (*A*) #24 is buccally rotated. Also note a severe labial inflammation on the #24 site. (*B*) After surgery. Connective tissue graft in conjunction with laterally rotating flap was a surgical choice for root coverage on this case. Note a thick labial tissue on both #23 and #25 sites allowed laterally rotating flap to cover up connective tissue graft (CTG) without recession on #23 and #25 site.

physically prevents the overgrowth of the gingiva and is often suggested for Down syndrome patients (**Figs. 11** and **12**).

Gingival Issues Relating to Orthodontics

Unerupted canines

Most commonly seen impacted teeth other than wisdom teeth are maxillary canines.[42] Only 33% of impacted canines are located labially.[43] Periapical radiographs, panoramic radiographs, and manual palpation can be the most basic and reliable methods of locating the impacted canines. Lately, the use of Cone Beam Computed Tomography (CBCT) cone beam technology allows very minimal radiation compared with a traditional spiral computed tomography (CT). Therefore, CBCT can be used as a diagnostic tool to evaluate an impacted tooth. Using CBCT technology can be a great help to determine the exact location of an impacted tooth and to rule out potential adjacent root resorption and the potential compromise in the periodontium associated with exposures (**Fig. 13**).

Labially positioned canines

Depending on the location of the impacted canines and the presence of attached gingiva, the following techniques are available[44]

Simple excision
Apically positioned flap/laterally sliding flap
Closed versus open eruption techniques

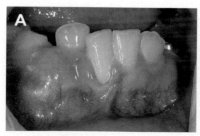 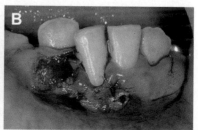

Fig. 9. (*A*) Preoperative picture of frenectomy and free gingival graft. (*B*) A graft was harvested from adjacent areas instead of palate.

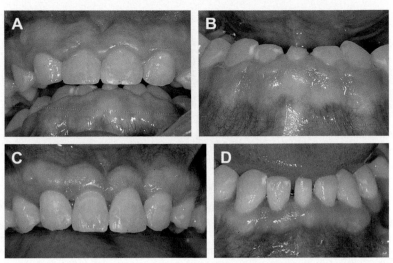

Fig. 10. (*A, B*) 18-year-old man with tetratology of Fallot, heart murmur, and deafness. Patient is taking a calcium channel blocker and a multivitamin. This is an example of DIGO. (*C, D*) Same patient 6 weeks after surgery. Note significant improvement in oral hygiene.

Table 1			
Drugs associated with DIGO			
Category	**Pharmacologic Agent**	**Trade Name**	**Prevalence**
Anticonvulsants	Phenytoin	Dilantin	50%[6,17,23]
	Sodium valproate (valproic acid)	Depakene, Depacon, Epilim.Valpro	Rare[2,5,23]
	Phenobarbitone	Phenobarbital, Donnatal	<5%[7]
	Vigabatrin	Sabril	Rare[8]
	Carbamazepine	Tegretol	None reported
Immunosuppressants	Cyclosporin	Neoral, Sandimmune	Adults 25%–30%[13,21,24] Children >70%[22]
Calcium channel blockers	Nifedipine	Adalat, Nifecard, Procardia, Tenif	6%–15%[18–20]
	Isradipine	DynaCirc	None reported
	Felodipine	Agon, Felodur, Lexxel, Plendil	Rare[2,20]
	Amlodipine	Lotrel, Norvasc	Rare[2,20]
	Verapamil	Calan, Covera, Isoptin, Tarka, Verelan	<5%[25]
	Diltiazem	Cardizem, Dilacor, Diltiamax, Tiazac	5%–20%[26]

Main categories of the drugs include anticonvulsants, immunosuppressants, and calcium channel blockers.

Adapted from Academy report: informational paper drug-associated gingival enlargement. J Periodontol 2004; with permission.

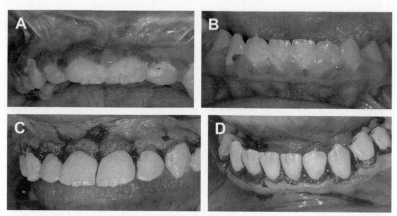

Fig. 11. (*A, B*) Patient with Noonan syndrome. Hypertrophic cardiomyopathy, pulmonary artery stenosis, ventricular septal defects, and valvular disorders are the main parts of congenital heart diseases. Most Noonan syndrome patients bruise easily and have bleeding disorders. Gingival hyperplasia with very poor oral hygiene. Patient stated, "it hurts to brush." (*C, D*) Immediate postoperative surgical picture. Internal and external beveling incisions were used to remove the excessive gingival tissue. Electrosurgery was also used to minimize the bleeding and cauterize.

One must consider the future mucogingival issues when exposing labially impacted canines. According to a study examining the long-term periodontal health of impacted canines, the conservative apical or lateral positioned flap showed better long-term outcome compared with a simple radical excision of tissue without considering attached tissue.[44]

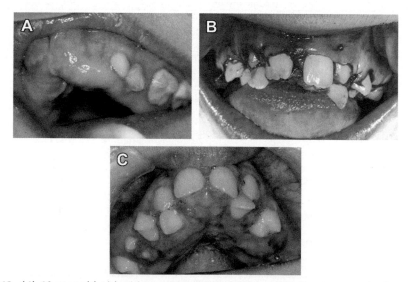

Fig. 12. (*A*) 10-year-old girl with prenatal exposure to cocaine. In utero cerebral vascular accident with hypoxic insult affecting basal ganglion and thalamus bilaterally. Patient is tracheostomy dependent. (*B*) Immediate postoperative photograph after gingivectomy/gingivoplasty. (*C*) 2 weeks followup. Teeth # 7 and 10 are planned for extractions.

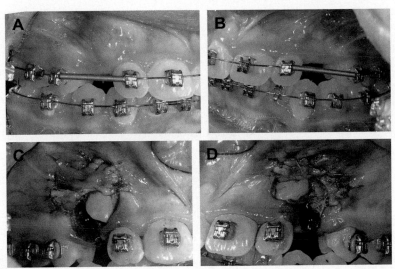

Fig. 13. (*A, B*) Pre-surgical pictures of missing # 6 and #11. (*C, D*) Immediate postoperative pictures. Once #6 was exposed, the flap was apically positioned and sutured. Likewise # 11 was exposed, and then the flap was slid laterally to ensure preservation of the labial gingival tissue.

A radical resection can lead to increased gingival recession and gingivitis due to lack of attached tissue.[45] At least 2 mm of attached gingiva apical to the canine is considered a must to avoid future gingival recession. In case it is absolutely impossible to rotate or apically position the attached tissue during surgical exposure, a free gingival graft is recommended to ensure a long-term gingival health and esthetic considerations.

Palatally positioned canines

Two different methods of exposures, open versus closed exposures, are available for palatally positioned canines. An open procedure recommends first uncovering the palatally impacted canines during the mixed dentition followed by orthodontic movements.[44] Surgically, open procedures uncover canines via removal of surrounding bone down to the Cemento Enamel Junction (CEJ), and the flap is repositioned with a keyhole opening. Once the canine erupts to the dental arch (in approximately 6–8 months) orthodontic forces are applied (**Figs. 14** and **15**).[44]

A closed exposure is more conventional and widely used. An orthodontic bracket or gold chain is placed on the day of the exposure surgery, typically with glass ionomer cement, and the orthodontic forces are applied.

Post-treatment study of the periodontal health of a closed technique subject showed higher root resorption on the lateral incisors and compromised bone levels on the interproximal surfaces of the lateral incisor and canines.[42] Another study suggests significantly improved long-term periodontal health and esthetic results on the canines exposed through the open technique.[45]

However, the result of systemic review indicates that there is no evidence to support one exposure method over the other[43] (50). In this author's opinion, perhaps the timing of the exposure and the earlier intervention of the impacted canine affect the overall improved results from the open exposure. Regardless of the exposure methods,

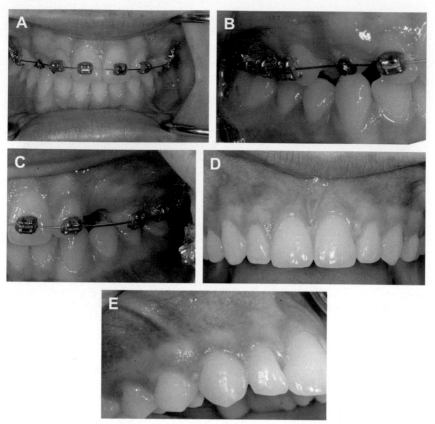

Fig. 14. (*A–C*) Prepalatal exposure pictures. Conventional closed technique was applied here with an orthodontic bracket applied on the day of surgical exposure. (*D, E*) 5-year postclose palatal exposure technique.

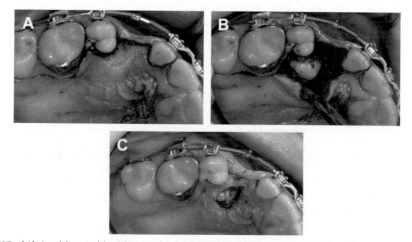

Fig. 15. (*A*) A midcrestal incision and sulcular incision around the #4 allow better access. (*B*) Canine #11 exposed and osteoplasty completed. (*C*) An access hole was created for the gold chain.

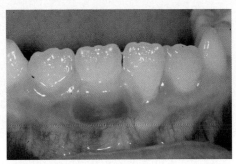

Fig. 16. 6-year-old healthy boy. The erythematous tissue did not respond to strick oral hygiene and chlorohexadine rinses. Excisional biopsy revealed a localized juvenile spongiotic hyperplasia.

plaque control and the tight communication between specialists (orthodontists, periodontists, oral surgeons, and pediatric dentists) are the keys to long-term success.

Localized juvenile spongiotic hyperplasia

This reactive process has been described as juvenile spongiotic gingivitis initially. When compared with pubertal gingivitis, this gingival disease is characterized by a lack of response to good oral hygiene and plaque control.[46]

It often presents in girls ages 5 to 11 undergoing orthodontics in anterior gingiva region.[47]

Diagnosis can be made by both clinical examination and hisopathological examination. Clinically, the lesions can range from a bright red granulation tissue to a simple exophytic papillary mass on the facial or interproximal areas. Treatment of choice is excision and re-evaluation. Most studies show a high recurrence rate from 6% to 16%.[46,47] The desired treatment outcomes are minimizing inflammation/localized infection, improving esthetics, and providing access for routine oral hygiene care (**Fig. 16**).

TRAUMA

Even in a radical situation as in trauma, preservation of dentition is the key to treating children. Too many times, esthetic disaster affects adults from a consequence of childhood trauma. Most often implants placed too early will have an ankylosed appearance (**Fig. 17**).

Unless children have a special concern such as ectodermal dysplasia or teeth agenesis, implants in children and adolescents must be avoided.

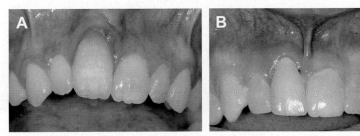

Fig. 17. (*A, B*) Examples of implants placed too early. Note an ankylosed appearance. (*A*) 29-year-old woman. (*B*) 34-year-old man. In both cases, crowns were replaced multiple times in attempts to improve and mask the underlying esthetic complications.

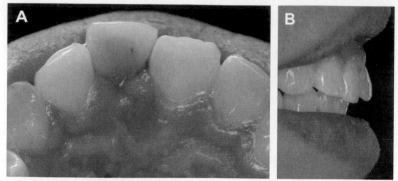

Fig. 18. (*A*, *B*) 17-year-old girl was referred to periodontist for the clinical crown lengthening procedure from a general dentist before crown procedure on #8. Previous history of trauma, and the tooth is treated with root canal and currently has a large build up. To avoid catastrophic esthetic failure, a combination of orthodontics and limited crown lengthening from the palatal approach will result in the most ideal outcome.

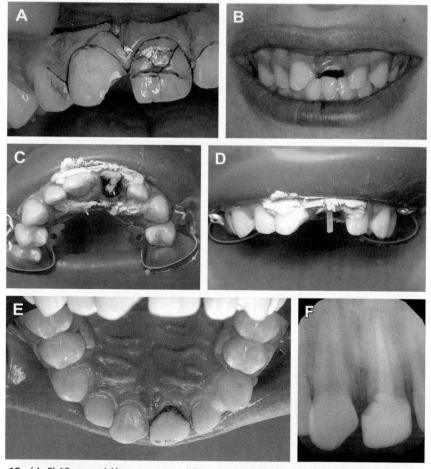

Fig. 19. (*A*, *B*) 13-year-old boy presents with trauma; patient fell in the bathtub. (*C–E*) Extensive build up on the #8 and #9 areas. (*F*) Root canal was completed on the #9. Instead of crown lengthening the #8 and #9 areas, orthodontic extrusion is recommended to increase ferrule in this case. Note patient's smile; it is considered gummy, showing excessive gingiva. (Special thanks to University of Washington Pediatric Dentistry department and Jane Steiber and Nestor Cohenca.)

Therefore, when teeth are traumatized and fractured, it is best to maintain the teeth until growth is completed in children. Although dental implants are a great replacement for lost and compromised teeth, when placed prematurely in growing children, adolescents, and young adults, they can lead to severe esthetic issues.

Alternatively, one must consider a clinical crown lengthening procedure to expose enough ferrule, or consider limited or full orthodontics to extrude the fractured pieces to at least temporarily maintain and restore teeth until more permanent solutions such as implants can be considered (**Figs. 18** and **19**).

SUMMARY

Regardless of the disease entity, prevention of tooth loss is the main objective of periodontal treatment in children. This article examined periodontal and gingival diseases and other issues relating to orthodontics such as impacted canines and inflammatory reactive gingival conditions. It also examined drug-induced gingival hyperplasia.

The author's experience mainly comes from hospital- and community-based dentistry. Frequently, socioeconomic status and the education levels of the patient's parents are different from that of the patients seen in private practice settings.

In summary, maintenance and preservation of teeth and prevention of tooth loss are the main desired outcomes of the periodontal treatment outlined in this article. Minimal treatment for the maximum result outlines the main philosophy behind pediatric periodontics. A team approach must be considered for success in treating children. Close communication with pediatric dentists and other specialists such as orthodontists, endodontists, and oral surgeons is key to a successful outcome.

ACKNOWLEDGMENTS

I would like to thank Dr Terry Thomas for immeasurable help and dedication on this manuscript.

REFERENCES

1. Loe H, Brown LJ. Early onset periodontitis in the United States of America. J Periodontol 1991;62:608–16.
2. Academy report position paper: periodontal disease in children and adolescents. 2003;74:1696–704.
3. Armitage G. Development of a classification system for periodontal diseases and conditions. Ann Periodontol 1999;4:1–6.
4. Waldrop TC, Anderson DC, Hallmon WW, et al. Periodontal manifestations of the heritable Mac-1, LFA-1, deficiency syndrome. J Periodontol 1987;58:400–16.
5. Meyle J. Leukocyte adhesion deficiency and prepubertal periodontitis. Periodontol 2000 1994;6:26–36.
6. Batista EL Jr, Novaes AB Jr, Calvano LM, et al. Necrotizing ulcerative periodontitis associated with severe congenital immunodeficiency in a prepubescent subject: clinical findings and response to intravenous immunoglobulin treatment. J Clin Periodontol 1999;26:499–504.
7. Plagmann HC, Kocher T, Kuhrau N, et al. Periodontal manifestation of hypophosphatasia. J Clin Periodontol 1994;21:710–6.
8. Dougherty N, Gataletto MA. Oral sequelae of chronic neutrophil defects: case report of a child with glycogen storage disease type 1b. Pediatr Dent 1995;17: 224–9.

9. Kamma JJ, Lygidakis NA, Nakou M, et al. Subgingival microflora and treatment in prepubertal periodontitis associated with chronic idiopathic neutropenia. J Clin Periodontol 1998;25:759–65.

10. Prichard JF, Ferguson DM, Windmiller J, et al. Prepubertal periodontitis affecting the deciduous dentition and permanent dentition in a patient with cyclic neutropenia. A case report and discussion. J Periodontol 1984;55:114–22.

11. Schroeder HE, Seger RA, Keller HU, et al. Behavior of neutrophilic granulocytes in a case of papillion lefevre syndrome. J Clin Periodontol 1983;10:618–35.

12. Tinanoff N, Tanzer JM, Kornman KS, et al. Treatment of the periodontal component of papillion lefevre syndrome. J Clin Periodontol 1986;13:6–10.

13. Izumi Y, Sugiyama S, Shinozuki O, et al. Defective neutrophil chemotaxis in Down's syndrome patients and its relationship to periodontal destruction. J Periodontol 1989;60:238–42.

14. Orner G. Periodontal disease among children with Down's syndrome and their siblings. J Dent Res 1976;55:778–82.

15. Mashimo PA, Yamamoto Y, Slots J, et al. The periodontal microflora of juvenile diabetes, culture, immunofluorescence, and serum antibody studies. J Periodontol 1983;54:420–30.

16. Periodontology AAP. Parameters of care on periodontics associated with systemic conditions. 2000;71:876–9.

17. Baer PN. The case for periodontosis as a clinical entitiy. J Periodontol 1971;42:516–20.

18. Periodontitis AAP. J Periodontol 2000;71:867–9.

19. Taiwo JO. Severity of necrotizing ulcerative gingivitis in Nigerian children. Periodontal Clin Investig 1995;17:24–7.

20. Conreas A, Falkler WA Jr, Enwonwu CO, et al. Human herpesviridae in acute necrotizing ulcerative gingivitis in children in Nigeria. Oral Microbiol Immunol 1997;12:259–65.

21. Loesche WJ, Syed SA, Laughon BE, et al. The bacteriology of acute necrotizing ulcerative gingivitis. J Periodontol 1982;53:223–30.

22. Johnson B, Engel D. A review of diagnosis, etiology and treatment. J Periodontol 1986;57:141–50.

23. Periodontology AAP. Parameter on mucogingival conditions. J Periodontol 2000;71:861–2.

24. Stoner JE, Mazdyasna S. Gingival recession in the lower incisor region of 15-year-old subjects. J Periodontol 1980;51(2):74–6.

25. Maynard JG Jr, Ochsenbein C. Mucogingival problems, prevalence and therapy in children. J Periodontol 1975;46(9):543–52.

26. Ochsenbein C, Maynard JG. The problem of attached gingiva in children. ASDC J Dent Child 1974;41(5):263–72.

27. Coatoam GW, Behrents RG, Bissada NF. The width of keratinized gingiva during orthodontic treatment: its significance and impact on periodontal status. J Periodontol 1981;52(6):307–13.

28. Ward VJ. A clinical assessment of the use of the free gingival graft for correcting localized recession associated with frenal pull. J Periodontol 1974;45(2):78–83.

29. Nabers JM. Free gingival grafts. Periodontics 1966;4(5):243–5.

30. Sullivan HC, Atkins JH. Free autogenous gingival grafts. I. Principles of successful grafting. Periodontics 1968;6(3):121–9.

31. Pasquinelli KL. The histology of new attachment utilizing a thick autogenous soft tissue graft in an area of deep recession: a case report. Int J Periodontics Restorative Dent 1995;15(3):248–57.

32. Hassell T, Page RC, Narayanan AS, et al. Diphenylhydantoin (Dilantin) gingival hyperplasia: drug induced abnormality of connective tissue. Proc Natl Acad Sci U S A 1976;73:2909–12.
33. Bolzani G, Della Coletta R, Martelli H Jr, et al. Cyclosporin A inhibits production and activity of matrix metalloproteinasese by gingival fibroblasts. J Periodontal Res 2000;35:51–8.
34. Marshall RI, Bartold PM. A Clinical review of drug induced gingival overgrowth. Aust Dent J 1999;44:219–32.
35. Somacarrera ML, Lucas M, Scully C, et al. Effectiveness of periodontal treatments on cyclosporine-induced gingival overgrowth in transplant patients. Br Dent J 1997;183:89–94.
36. Khocht A, Schneider LC. Periodontal management of gingival overgrowth in the heart transplant patient: a case review. J Periodonto 1997;68(11):1140–6.
37. Payne VM. Periodontal management of gingival overgrowth in the heart transplant patient: a case report. J Periodontol 1998;69:1314–5.
38. Gomez E, Sánchez-Nuñez M, Sanchez JE, et al. Treatment of cyclosporin-induced gingival hyperplasia with azithromycin. Nephrol Dial Transplant 1997; 12:2694–7.
39. Stachan D, Burton I, Pearson GJ. Is oral azithromycin effective for the treatment of cyclosporin-induced gingival hyperplasia in cardiac transplant recipients? J Clin Pharm Ther 2003;28:329–38.
40. Marshall RI, Bartold PM. A clinical review of drug induced gingival overgrowth. Oral Surg Oral Med Oral Pathol 1993;76:543–8.
41. Ilgenli T, Atilla G, Baylas H. Effectiveness of periodontal therapy in patients with drug induced gingival overgrowth. Long term results. J Periodontol 1999;70: 967–72.
42. Woloshyn H, Artun J, Kennedy DB, et al. Pulpal and periodontal reactions to orthodontic alignment of palatally impacted canines. Angle Orthod 1994;64: 257–64.
43. Johnston WD. Treatment of palatally impacted canine teeth. Am J Orthod 1969; 51:30–40.
44. Tegsjo T, Valerius-Olsson H, Andersson L. Periodontal conditions following surgical exposure of unerupted maxillary canines—a long term follow-up study of two surgical techniques. Swed Dent J 1984;8(6):257–63.
45. Schmidt A, Kokich VG. Periodontal response to early uncovering, autonomous eruption, and orthodontic alignment of palatally impacted maxillary canines. Am J Orthod Dentofacial Orthop 2007;131:449–55.
46. Darling MR, Daley TD, Wilson A, et al. Juvenile spongiotic gingivitis. J Periodontol 2007;78(7):1235–40.
47. Chang JY, Kessler HP, Wright JM. Localized juvenile spongiotic gingival hyperplasia. Oral Surg Oral Med Oral Pathol 2008;106(3):411–8.

Overview of Trauma Management for Primary and Young Permanent Teeth

Dennis J. McTigue, DDS, MS

KEYWORDS

- Dental injuries • Traumatic injuries • Avulsion • Luxation • Intrusion
- Crown fractures • Root fractures

KEY POINTS

- Falls are the most frequent cause of dental trauma among preschool and school-age children. Sports-related injuries and altercations are more common in adolescents. Dental trauma may be an indication of child abuse.
- Dental injuries are a subset of head trauma. The history in children with dental trauma should include the time, place, and mechanism of the injury and a thorough neurologic history.
- Avulsed primary teeth should not be reimplanted.
- Avulsed permanent teeth should be reimplanted immediately by the first capable person (eg, the injured child, a parent, teacher, coach, neighbor.) If immediate replantation is not possible the tooth should be stored in cold milk or in a cup with the child's saliva. It should not be stored in water.

Managing injuries to children's teeth in the primary and early mixed dentitions can be challenging. Injured children and their parents are often anxious and this can complicate the provision of prompt, appropriate care. The clinician must be able to assess the injury, prioritize treating those problems that require immediate attention, and minimize the child's fear and anxiety.

An excellent online resource for current treatment guidelines is *The Dental Trauma Guide* (http://www.dentaltraumaguide.org).[1] This guide, developed by Dr Jens O. Andreasen and sponsored in part by the University Hospital, Copenhagen and the International Association for Dental Traumatology (IADT), contains updated guidelines on a broad array of dental injuries and is easy to use.

EPIDEMIOLOGY AND CAUSE

Differences in study design and sampling criteria make precise estimates of the incidence and prevalence of dental injuries difficult to determine. Up to 40% of preschool

Division of Pediatric Dentistry and Community Oral Health, College of Dentistry, Ohio State University, 305 West 12th Avenue, Columbus, OH 43210, USA
E-mail address: Mctigue.1@osu.edu

Dent Clin N Am 57 (2013) 39–57
http://dx.doi.org/10.1016/j.cden.2012.09.005
0011-8532/13/$ – see front matter © 2013 Elsevier Inc. All rights reserved.

children suffer injuries to their primary teeth, with the peak incidence occurring in the toddler stages (2 to 3 years), when young children are developing their mobility skills.[2,3] Falls during play account for most injuries to young permanent teeth.[4] Children who participate in contact sports are at greater risk for dental trauma, although the use of mouth guards reduces their frequency. Automobile accidents cause many dental injuries in the teenage years, particularly when occupants not wearing seatbelts hit the steering wheel or dashboard. Many apparently minor dental injuries go unreported, so it is safe to assume that up to half of all children suffer some dental trauma.

Maxillary central incisors are the most commonly injured teeth, followed by the maxillary lateral incisors and the mandibular incisors. The ability of the upper lip to protect the maxillary teeth is affected by the degree of prominence of the anterior teeth (**Fig. 1**). The normal horizontal distance between the maxillary and mandibular incisors (overjet) is between 1 and 3 mm. Overjets greater than 4 mm increase the likelihood of dental trauma by 2 to 3 times.[5,6]

Dental trauma may be an important clinical marker for child abuse, because up to 50% to 75% of all cases involve some form of orofacial injury.[7]

Potential signs of child abuse include:

- Bruises in various stages of healing indicating multiple traumatic incidents
- Torn upper labial frena
- Bruising of the labial sulcus in young, preambulatory patients
- Bruising on the soft tissues of the cheek.

EVALUATION
History

Knowing when, where, and how the injury occurred assists the clinician in determining the severity of the injury. The time that has elapsed since the injury took place affects the treatment and, in most cases, the prognosis. Knowledge regarding the mechanism of injury helps to determine the severity of the injury and the risk of associated injuries. A thorough neurologic history should be obtained, because dental injuries are a subset of head trauma.[8] The patient should be promptly referred for medical evaluation of a potential closed head injury if any of the following signs are present:

- Dizziness
- Headache

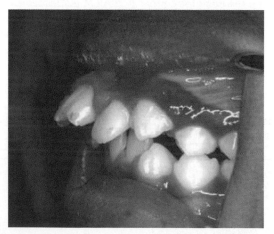

Fig. 1. A large horizontal overjet increases the risk for dental injury.

- Nausea/vomiting
- Loss of memory
- Loss of consciousness
- Lethargy or irritability

As noted earlier, the possibility of child abuse also must be considered. The child's medical history should be obtained, with particular attention given to medications, drug allergies, and status of tetanus immunization.

Clinical Examination

A thorough clinical examination should include an assessment of:

- The facial skeleton to determine discontinuities of facial bones. Extraoral wounds and bruises should be recorded. The temporomandibular joints should be palpated, and any swelling, clicking, or crepitus should be noted. Mandibular function in all excursive movements should be checked. Any stiffness or pain in the child's neck necessitates immediate referral to a physician to rule out cervical spine injury.
- Intraoral and extraoral soft tissues, including the lips, frena, tongue, gingivae, oral mucosa, and palate.
- All teeth (anterior and posterior), to rule out fractures, discoloration, displacements, pulp exposures, and increased mobility. Fractures of the posterior teeth may occur after trauma to the chin and are associated with fractures of the mandibular condyles and cervical spine.
- Does the child have spontaneous pain in any teeth as a result of the injury? This pain may indicate pulpal exposure or inflammation.
- Are any of the teeth tender to touch or the pressure of eating? This symptom indicates periodontal ligament (PDL) damage or displacement.
- Are any of the teeth sensitive to hot or cold? This symptom may indicate pulp exposure or inflammation.
- Is there a change in the child's bite or occlusion? This change indicates displaced teeth or possibly a facial fracture.

Radiographic Examination

Radiographs enable the clinician to gather information needed for an accurate diagnosis and plan of treatment. They are useful to determine the

- Extent of root development
- Position of unerupted teeth
- Size of pulp chambers
- Relationship between the injured primary teeth and their permanent successors
- Periapical radiolucencies
- Root fractures
- Extent and type of root resorption
- Degree of tooth displacement
- Jaw fractures
- Presence of tooth fragments and other foreign bodies in soft tissues

Baseline radiographs at the initial appointment are important even if they seem to show negative findings, because they can be compared with subsequent radiographic evidence at follow-up appointments.

Radiographic techniques

All images should clearly show the apical areas of traumatized teeth. The guidelines of the IADT call for multiple images taken from slightly different angles both vertically and horizontally to verify the location and extent of a pathologic condition.[9] Standard anterior occlusal views are appropriate to detect injuries to primary incisors. A lateral anterior view can also be helpful to determine the relationship between an intruded primary tooth and its developing permanent successor (**Fig. 2**). Exposure times vary depending on the equipment used, but doubling the exposure time is usually sufficient for this view. Film/sensor holding devices should be used to expose periapical images of injured permanent teeth to enable duplication of the same views at subsequent visits. The presence of foreign bodies such as tooth fragments in the lips or tongue can be detected by reducing the normal exposure time. The film or sensor is placed beneath the tissue to be examined, and the radiograph is exposed.

Timing of follow-up radiographs

Many pathologic changes are not immediately apparent in radiographs. It takes approximately 3 weeks to detect periapical radiolucencies that are caused by pulpal necrosis, and inflammatory root resorption may also be evident at this time. After approximately 6 to 7 weeks, replacement resorption, or ankylosis, can be seen. Thus, there is adequate rationale to obtain postoperative radiographs at 1 month after the injury. In the absence of any clinical signs or symptoms, such as development of swelling, fistula, mobility, tooth discoloration, or pain, additional films are not indicated until 6 months after the injury. If changes are to appear radiographically, they usually do so by this time.

CLASSIFICATION OF DENTOALVEOLAR INJURIES
Fractures

Trauma to the mouth may cause fractures of the teeth or damage to the supporting alveolar bone and periodontium. Fractures of the crown are classified as complicated (involving the neurovascular pulp) or uncomplicated (involving only the enamel or the enamel and dentin). Horizontal, vertical, and oblique fractures of the root also occur.

Luxation Injuries

Luxation injuries involve the supporting structures of the teeth, including the PDL and alveolar bone. The primary goal in the treatment of luxation injuries is to maintain the

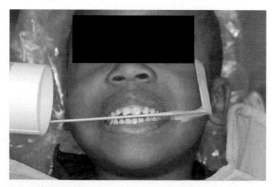

Fig. 2. Lateral anterior radiograph.

vitality of the PDL, which supports the tooth in its socket. Luxation injuries are classified as follows:

- Concussion: the tooth is neither loose nor displaced; it may be tender with the pressure of biting because of inflammation of the PDL.
- Subluxation: the tooth is loose but not displaced from its socket. The PDL fibers are damaged and inflamed.
- Intrusion: the tooth is driven into the socket, compressing the PDL and fracturing the alveolar socket.
- Extrusion: the tooth is centrally dislocated from its socket; the PDL is lacerated and inflamed.
- Lateral luxation: the tooth is displaced anteriorly, posteriorly, or laterally; the PDL is lacerated and the supporting bone is fractured.
- Avulsion: the tooth is completely displaced from the alveolar ridge; the PDL is severed and fracture of the alveolus may occur.

PATHOLOGIC SEQUELAE OF TRAUMA TO TEETH

Complications after traumatic injuries to teeth may appear shortly after the injury (eg, infection of the PDL or dark discoloration of the crown) or after several months (eg, yellow discoloration of the crown and external root resorption). It is not possible to accurately identify the histopathologic condition of a dental pulp based on clinical symptoms. The following terms describe a spectrum of clinical signs and symptoms that accompany inflammation and degeneration of the pulp or PDL.

Pulpitis

Pulpitis is the initial response of the tooth to trauma and it accompanies almost every injury. Signs include sensitivity to percussion and capillary congestion, which may be clinically apparent from the lingual surface of the tooth using transillumination. Pulpitis may be reversible in minor injuries or may progress to irreversible pulpitis and pulp necrosis.

Pulp Necrosis

Injured pulps may lose their vitality either because of damage to the vascular tissue at the apex and the resulting ischemia or because of necrosis of exposed coronal pulp tissue. If the necrotic pulp becomes infected with oral microorganisms either because of luxation of the root and ingress through the lacerated PDL or via an exposed pulp, pain and root resorption can occur. In the primary dentition, extraction is indicated to prevent damage to the permanent successor. A pulpectomy is indicated in the permanent dentition. When the necrotic pulp is not infected, it may remain asymptomatic, both clinically and radiographically.

Tooth Discoloration

Injuries to the primary incisors frequently cause tooth discoloration (**Fig. 3**). Blood vessels within the pulp chamber can rupture, depositing blood pigment in the dentinal tubules. This blood may resorb completely or can persist to some degree throughout the life of the tooth. Teeth that discolor are not necessarily necrotic, particularly when the color change occurs within a few days of the injury.[10] However, primary teeth with dark discoloration that persists for months after the injury are likely to be necrotic, but may remain asymptomatic. So, in healthy children, tooth color alone does not dictate treatment of primary incisors. Other signs or symptoms of infection, like periapical radiolucency, pain, swelling, parulis, or increased mobility, should be detected before

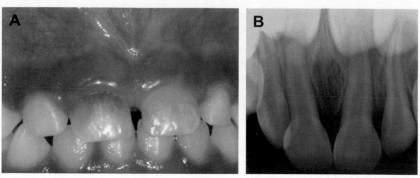

Fig. 3. Tooth discoloration. (*A*) Discolored primary incisor. (*B*) No radiographic evidence of disease associated with the discolored tooth.

the tooth is extracted. In the permanent dentition, persistent, dark discoloration indicates that pulp necrosis is likely and a pulpectomy is indicated.

A yellowish discoloration of both primary and permanent teeth may occur if they undergo pulp canal obliteration (PCO).

PCO

PCO is a common finding in luxated primary incisors, particularly when the injury occurred before completion of the root development of the tooth. It is also associated with luxation injuries to permanent incisors, and, again, is most common in those with incomplete root development (**Fig. 4**).[11] The entire pulp chamber and canal appear radiopaque in radiographs and the crown may have a yellowish color. The process of accelerated dentinal apposition in PCO is not well understood, but primary teeth with PCO tend to resorb normally. Pulp necrosis is rare in teeth with PCO and root canal treatment is rarely indicated in either the primary or permanent dentitions.

Inflammatory Resorption

Inflammatory resorption can occur internally or externally. It is related to an infected pulp and an inflamed PDL. It can resorb roots quickly and, in the primary dentition, this inflammatory process can damage developing teeth, so extraction of the offending tooth is indicated. In the permanent dentition, inflammatory resorption can be radiologically evident within several weeks of an injury (**Fig. 5**). It is treated by removing the pulp and applying calcium hydroxide.

Replacement Resorption

Replacement resorption results after irreversible injury to the PDL. Alveolar bone directly contacts and becomes fused with the root surface, causing ankylosis. These teeth have no physiologic mobility and have a dull, metallic sound when percussed. As the child grows, alveolar bone undergoes normal physiologic osteoclastic and osteoblastic activity, replacing the root with bone (**Fig. 6**).

Injuries to Developing Teeth

The proximity of the apices of primary incisors to the developing tooth buds of their permanent successors creates a potential for damage to the latter when the former are injured. The greatest risk for injuries to permanent teeth exists when the primary teeth are intruded or avulsed and before the age of 3 years, when the permanent tooth

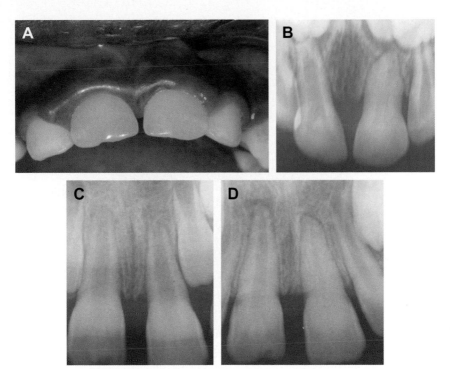

Fig. 4. (A) The maxillary left primary central incisor shows yellow discoloration. (B) Radiograph indicates PCO of that tooth. (C) Immediate postoperative radiograph of a luxated, immature permanent incisor (number 9). (D) 18-month postoperative radiograph showing PCO in tooth number 9.

crowns are calcifying. White or yellow-brown discoloration is the most common deformity, but enamel hypoplasia, crown and root dilacerations, and ectopic or delayed eruption have all been reported (**Fig. 7**).

TREATMENT
Primary Dentition Injuries

The most important consideration in managing injured primary teeth should be the well-being of the developing permanent successors. Parents should be thoroughly informed of the intimate relationship between the apex of the primary incisor and the developing permanent tooth bud. The benefits of saving an injured primary tooth versus the potential risk of damage to the developing permanent tooth should be explained and documented. This understanding is integral to acquiring valid informed consent from a distraught parent requesting relatively heroic measures to save an injured primary tooth.

Luxation injuries
Luxation injuries involve damage to the PDL and are the most common injuries in the primary dentition. This situation is because the supporting tissues in young children are pliable and allow the teeth to move, frequently without fracturing.

Concussion
A concussion injury transmits the force of the blow to the PDL but causes no mobility. The only clinical sign is tenderness to percussion. Treatment is rarely needed, but

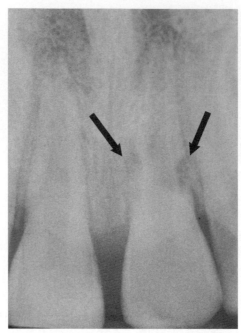

Fig. 5. Inflammatory resorption destroying the root of this recently luxated permanent incisor (*arrows*).

adjusting the occlusion may relieve symptoms in a hypersensitive child. The concussed tooth should be monitored for several months to rule out potential complications.

Subluxation

The subluxed tooth has increased mobility but is not displaced from its socket. Sulcular bleeding may be present. Parents are instructed to keep the area clean and to

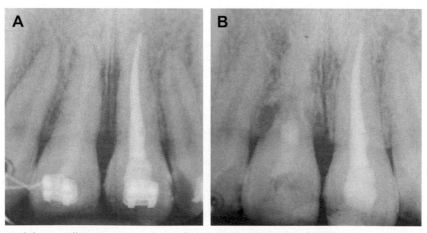

Fig. 6. (*A*) Immediate postoperative radiograph showing calcium hydroxide paste in tooth number 8, which had been avulsed and replanted after 90 minutes. (*B*) One-year postoperative radiograph showing replacement resorption of tooth number 8.

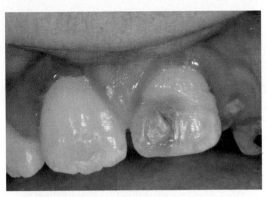

Fig. 7. Permanent incisor damaged secondary to trauma to its primary predecessor.

have the child avoid incising on the involved teeth for 2 weeks. This is a common injury in the primary dentition, and normal function returns in most cases, although close monitoring for pathologic sequelae is indicated.

Lateral luxation
This is a more serious injury, with the tooth displaced out of its normal position, frequently in a palatal direction. Radiographs are indicated to rule out root fractures and to indicate the position of the root in the alveolus. If the tooth is not interfering with the occlusion it may be allowed to reposition spontaneously. Some investigators recommend that when occlusal interference does occur the tooth should be manually repositioned and splinted for 2 to 3 weeks. However, because of the increased risk of pulpal necrosis and the potential for damage to the developing permanent successor, this author recommends extracting severely displaced primary incisors.

Intrusion
Intrusion of a primary incisor implies a high risk of damage to the permanent successor, and the injured child's parents should be so advised at the time of injury. Conservative treatment is indicated, because damage to the permanent tooth bud can occur during extraction of the intruded primary incisor. A lateral anterior radiograph is taken to determine the position of the intruded primary incisor relative to the developing tooth bud (see **Figs. 2** and **8**). Most intruded incisors are displaced labially and away from the tooth bud. These incisors are allowed to reerupt spontaneously, anticipating that most survive without complications. If the intruded tooth impinges on the developing tooth bud, it is carefully extracted, with the forceps gently engaged on the mesial and distal surfaces of the tooth. Most intruded primary incisors partially or completely reerupt within 4 to 5 months.

Extrusion
The extruded tooth is displaced centrally from its socket and has increased mobility. Radiographs should be taken to rule out other injuries. Treatment is determined by the degree of extrusion, mobility, and the child's ability to cope with treatment. Minor extrusions can be repositioned, whereas severe extrusions should be extracted.

Avulsion
Avulsed primary incisors should not be replanted because of the risk of damage to the permanent successors.[12] Radiographs are indicated to confirm that the tooth is not intruded. Losing anterior primary teeth is often more traumatic for the parents than

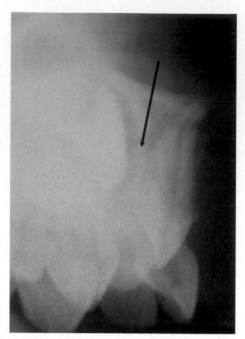

Fig. 8. Lateral anterior radiograph showing lack of contact between intruded primary incisor and the developing permanent successor (*arrow*).

it is for the injured child, and the clinician must thoroughly explain the rationale against replantation. Once the primary canines have erupted, there is little concern about loss of space in the anterior segment with early loss of primary incisors. If esthetics is a major concern, a fixed or removable partial denture can be fabricated.

Crown Fractures

Any blow that causes a tooth to fracture is likely to cause a luxation injury as well. The clinician is advised to carefully examine all fractured teeth and to manage associated luxation injuries as explained earlier.

Uncomplicated crown fractures

These fractures include the enamel only or enamel and dentin but without a pulp exposure. Periapical radiographs are indicated to rule out other injuries and to assess the degree of physiologic root resorption. In minor fractures, the sharp edges can be smoothed with sandpaper disks or finishing burs. In larger fractures including the incisal angle, adhesive resin-based composite restorations or preveneered stainless steel crowns may be indicated.[13]

Complicated crown fractures

These injuries involve a pulp exposure, and treatment is predicated on the life expectancy of the tooth and the child's behavior. In young children with immature roots (younger than 3 years), a pulpotomy is indicated to preserve the pulp vitality in the root. When the root is mature, a complete pulpectomy with a resorbable paste like zinc oxide and eugenol may be performed. Treatment of complicated crown fractures should be completed as soon as practical after the injury, usually within 1 or 2 days. As noted earlier, the child must be controlled to complete the pulpal therapy and to restore the tooth, often indicating sedation or protective stabilization.

Crown/root fractures
Primary teeth with fractures that extend through the crown to the root should be extracted. A radiograph is indicated to assess the degree of damage. To avoid injuring the developing tooth bud, root fragments should be left to resorb spontaneously if they cannot be extracted easily.

Root fractures
When primary roots fracture in the apical third, the coronal fragment may not be displaced and may have adequate stability to allow its retention in the mouth. If the coronal fragment is displaced, it should be extracted and the apical fragment left to resorb spontaneously.

Permanent Dentition Injuries

Luxation injuries
Luxation injuries of permanent teeth are true dental emergencies. Management of these injuries focuses on maintaining the vitality of the PDL, and immediate management is necessary to achieve the best possible outcome.

Concussion
No treatment is usually indicated, but the involved teeth can be taken out of occlusion if the child complains of pain. The prognosis is good, but pulp necrosis and root resorption have been reported, so close follow-up is advised.

Subluxation
Subluxation injuries must be followed carefully, because the prognosis for survival of pulp in mature permanent teeth is significantly worse than in primary teeth. Radiographic monitoring beginning at 4 weeks and continuing up to a year is recommended to rule out pulp necrosis and inflammatory resorption. Immature teeth with open apices are less likely to undergo pulp necrosis but more likely to undergo PCO. A light splint for 2 weeks may be indicated for subluxated teeth if the patient requires it for comfort.[9]

Intrusion
Intrusion injuries in permanent teeth are difficult to manage and have a poor prognosis for healing. Pulpal necrosis, root resorption, and alveolar bone loss are common sequelae, and treatment is controversial because of the lack of clinical research. Recent IADT guidelines recommend different strategies depending on the apical development of the intruded tooth.[9]

Immature teeth (open apices, thin root walls) that are intruded less than 7 mm are allowed to re-emerge spontaneously. Orthodontic repositioning using light forces should be used if no movement is noted within 3 weeks. Immature teeth intruded more than 7 mm should be orthodontically or surgically repositioned (**Fig. 9**).

Mature permanent teeth (closed apices, thickened root walls) that are intruded less than 3 mm should be allowed to re-emerge without intervention. If no movement is noted within 2 weeks, they should be repositioned surgically or orthodontically before they ankylose. These teeth intruded beyond 3 mm should be repositioned surgically. Prophylactic pulpectomy with placement of calcium hydroxide (CaOH) is indicated within 3 weeks, because pulp necrosis and inflammatory resorption are likely in this injury. Obturation with gutta percha can occur after 1 to 2 months if signs of root

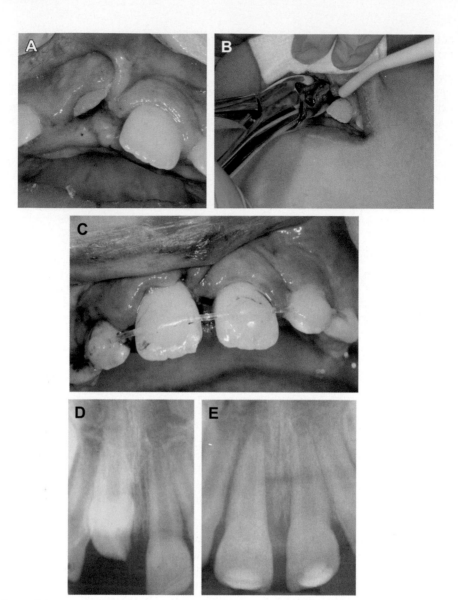

Fig. 9. (*A*) Permanent incisor intruded approximately 10 mm. (*B*) Surgical repositioning of intruded teeth with forceps. (*C*) Tooth repositioned and splint applied. (*D*) Preoperative radiograph. (*E*) Postoperative radiograph.

resorption do not present, but radiographic monitoring of the tooth should continue for at least 1 year.

Extrusion and lateral luxation

Luxation injuries in which the teeth are extruded or laterally displaced must be reduced so that the tooth is returned to its normal position and does not interfere with occlusion. Profound local aesthesia is indicated, and the tooth should be repositioned within 2 hours to favor optimal healing. A light splint is applied for 2 to 3 weeks, gingival lacerations are sutured, and chlorhexidine mouth rinse is prescribed.[9] In mature teeth, a CaOH pulpectomy is completed, and gutta percha obturation follows after 1 month if no root resorption occurs. Immature teeth with open apices have a chance to revascularize and maintain their vitality, so the decision to initiate therapy should be delayed until clinical or radiographic signs indicate necrosis.

Avulsion

The prognosis for survival of an avulsed permanent tooth is indirectly related to the amount of time spent out of the tooth socket. Maintaining PDL vitality is crucial to healing and more than 90% of avulsed teeth are saved if replanted within 5 minutes. The chances of success decrease to near zero if the tooth is stored dry for more than an hour. So it is critical that the avulsed permanent tooth is replanted as soon as possible (preferably at the site of injury) by the first capable person (eg, the injured child, a parent, teacher, coach, or pediatrician).[14]

Replantation technique

- Hold the tooth carefully by the crown to prevent damage to the PDL (**Fig. 10**).
- Remove debris by gentle rinsing with saline or tap water; no attempt should be made to sterilize or scrub the tooth.
- Manually replant the tooth in its socket as soon as possible.
- Apply a light, functional splint for 2 weeks.
- Complete a CaOH pulpectomy after 1 week.

Tooth transport solutions

Immediate replantation is not always possible. The vitality of PDL cells may be preserved by storing the tooth in a physiologic storage medium like Hanks balanced salt solution (HBSS), which supplies the tooth with inorganic ions and maintains a physiologic pH and osmotic pressure. HBSS may be purchased in an avulsed tooth preservation system called Save-A-Tooth (Phoenix-Lazerus, Pottstown, PA) (**Fig. 10A**). The use of such a system, even for several hours, increases the likelihood of survival of the PDL.

Cold milk is the best alternative storage medium for avulsed teeth if HBSS is not available. Milk is readily available and relatively aseptic, and Its osmolality is more conducive to maintaining the vitality of the PDL than is saline solution or tap water. Extraoral storage of avulsed teeth is improved by using chilled storage media. The avulsed tooth should be placed in a container of milk that is packed in ice, which maintains the cold temperature without diluting the milk and decreasing its osmolality.

Saliva is an alternative if milk or HBSS are not available immediately. The tooth should be placed into a container of the child's saliva. Holding the tooth in the child's mouth is not advised because it can be further traumatized, swallowed, or aspirated. Tap water should not be used because its low osmolality causes the cells to rupture within minutes.

Splinting technique

A variety of splinting techniques are available, but the author favors the use of 22.67-kg (50- lb) monofilament fishing line tacked to the teeth with composite resin (see **Figs. 9C** and **10D**). It is inexpensive, readily available, and functions well. A light orthodontic wire can also work, and several commercial products are also available. The ideal splint should:

1. Be passive and not apply force to the tooth
2. Be flexible and allow functional movement of the tooth
3. Allow for vitality testing and endodontic access
4. Be easy to apply and remove

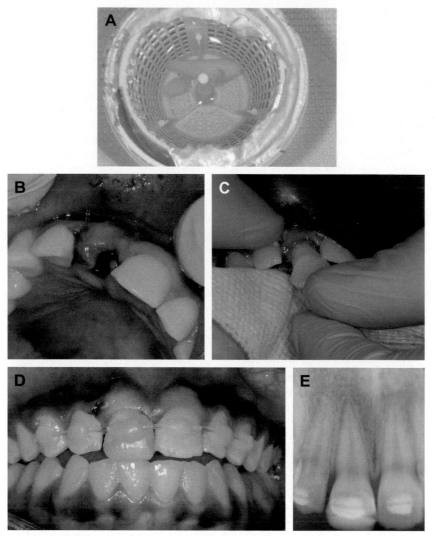

Fig. 10. Tooth replantation technique. (*A*) Avulsed tooth stored in Save-A-Tooth. (*B*) Tooth socket. (*C*) Tooth gently replanted in socket. (*D*) Tooth repositioned and splint applied. (*E*) Radiograph showing tooth appropriately repositioned.

Crown Fractures

Most fractures of the permanent teeth, even those with exposure of pulp, can be treated successfully hours after the injury, depending on the level of inflammation and vitality of the pulp. However, to optimize comfort and functional and cosmetic outcomes, the child should be treated as soon as possible.

Enamel and Dentin Fractures

Teeth with fractures that involve only the enamel or the enamel and dentin can readily be restored soon after the injury. Sealing exposed dentin with a bonding agent enables the unexposed pulp to form reparative dentin. A glass ionomer liner is placed over any exposed dentin followed by a dentin bonding agent. The tooth is then restored with an acid-etch/composite resin technique. If adequate time is not available to restore the tooth completely, an interim covering of resin material (a resin patch) can be used as a temporary seal until a final restoration can be placed.

Tooth fragments from crown fractures can be reattached if they are retrieved and kept properly hydrated (**Fig. 11**).[15] Special solutions are not necessary, because they have no fibroblasts to keep viable. However, the fragment should be kept hydrated in tap water, because discoloration occurs with desiccation. The fractured tooth can be restored with composite resin materials if the fragment is not retrieved.

FRACTURES INVOLVING THE PULP

Managing crown fractures that expose the pulp is particularly challenging. The treatment varies based on the vitality of the pulp and the maturation of the root. Importantly, the lack of an adequate seal can lead to failure. In immature teeth, the objective is to preserve pulp vitality to enable physiologic maturation of the root. Maintaining pulp vitality is also desirable in mature teeth but is not critical to the long-term prognosis, because the root apices are closed and the root walls are thickened. So the clinician may elect to complete gutta percha obturations on these teeth.

Criteria for Successful Pulp Therapy

Criteria for successful pulp therapy include the following:

1. Completion of root development in immature teeth
2. Absence of clinical signs such as pain, mobility, or fistula
3. Absence of radiographic signs of pathologic processes, such as periapical radiolucency of bone or root resorption

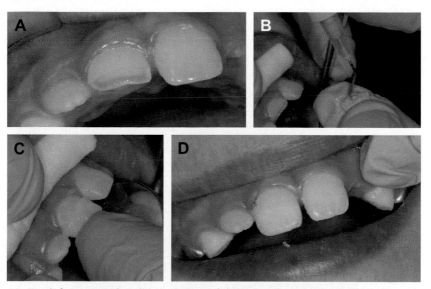

Fig. 11. Tooth fragment rebonding technique. (*A*) Uncomplicated fracture of tooth number 8. (*B*) After acid-etching and bonding, composite resin is applied to coronal fragment that had its dentin slightly trenched to accommodate the material. (*C*) Fragment repositioned. (*D*) Final finish.

Three treatment alternatives are available for exposed pulps:

1. Direct pulp cap
2. Pulpotomy
3. Pulpectomy

DIRECT PULP CAP

The direct pulp cap is indicated for small exposures in mature teeth that can be treated soon after an injury.[9] Ideally, the pulp is minimally inflamed and not contaminated with debris. The tooth is isolated and gently cleaned with water. CaOH paste or mineral trioxide aggregate (MTA) is applied directly to the pulp tissue and to surrounding dentin. An acid-etch/composite resin system is appropriate for the initial restoration, and it is critical that the tooth is sealed to prevent further contamination by oral bacteria. A calcific bridge stimulated by the capping material should be evident radiographically in 2 to 3 months.

A direct cap is not indicated in fractures exposing pulps of immature permanent teeth with incomplete root development. If the treatment fails and the pulp becomes necrotic, the root ceases its development and remains immature, with thin dentinal walls. The preferred treatment in pulp exposures of immature permanent teeth is pulpotomy.

PULPOTOMY

The successful pulpotomy technique removes only the inflamed pulp tissue and leaves healthy tissue to enhance physiologic maturation of the root. Cvek[16] reported that in most cases of pulps exposed for more than a few hours inflammation rarely extended beyond 2 mm, and conservative removal of this tissue is the treatment of choice (**Fig. 12**).

The tooth is isolated and the inflamed pulp is gently removed to a level approximately 2 mm below the exposure site with a sterile bur at high speed. Copious irrigation is essential to avoid pulp injury. CaOH or MTA pulp dressing is gently placed into the preparation covered by glass ionomer lining. Again, a bacteria-tight coronal seal is essential for the success. The tooth can then be esthetically restored with composite resin.

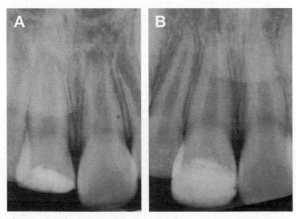

Fig. 12. (*A*) Immediate postoperative radiograph of immature permanent incisor (number 8) after partial pulpotomy (Cvek) technique. (*B*) 3-year postoperative radiograph showing physiologic maturation of tooth number 8 with apical closure and root wall thickening.

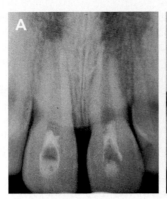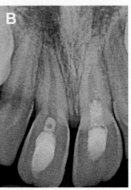

Fig. 13. Revascularization of necrotic immature permanent incisors. (*A*) Initial treatment radiograph showing open apices. (*B*) 2-year postoperative radiograph showing completion of root development.

PULPECTOMY

A pulpectomy completely removes pulp tissue from the crown and root and is indicated in mature teeth when no vital tissue remains or when the permanent restoration requires a post buildup. In the absence of inflammatory root resorption, treatment is to obturate the canal with gutta percha.

Treating a nonvital immature tooth with an open apex is one of the greatest challenges facing the clinician. Physiologic root maturation cannot occur with a necrotic pulp and traditional apexification procedures with CaOH have not proved to ensure long-term success.

An apical barrier technique with MTA is an option for managing devitalized immature incisors.[17,18] The material is placed at the apex and, after it sets, the root is filled with gutta percha. Although successful, this treatment still yields shortened roots and thin walls, leaving the tooth at risk for subsequent cervical root fracture. Regenerative endodontic procedures present the best option for long-term success in treating necrotic, immature teeth.

Regenerative Endodontics

Regenerative endodontic procedures seek to restore normal physiologic function by replacing damaged dentin, root structures, and pulp cells with live tissues (**Fig. 13**).[19] The root canal system is disinfected and bleeding is stimulated from the apical papilla to fill the root chamber with a blood clot.[20] Growth factors in the area then act on dental stem cells and differentiate into healthy cells of the pulp-dentin complex that can complete physiologic root maturation.

No evidence-based guidelines are available in the emerging field of regenerative endodontics to guide the clinician regarding its precise indications or technique.[21] The technique will be further refined with more research and this will lead to its greater use in the future.

SUMMARY AND RECOMMENDATIONS

- The Dental Trauma Guide at http://www.dentaltraumaguide.org is an online resource for current guidelines on managing dental trauma.
- Almost half of all children suffer injuries to their teeth. Falls are the most frequent cause of dental trauma among preschool and school-age children.

Sports-related injuries and accidents are more common in adolescents. Dental trauma may be an indication of child abuse.

- Treatment priorities for injured primary teeth include adequate pain control, safe management of the child's behavior, and protection of the developing permanent teeth. Avulsed primary incisors should not be replanted.
- Luxated permanent teeth should be managed as soon as possible. Intruded teeth can be left to re-emerge or be repositioned depending on their root development and amount of intrusion.
- Avulsed permanent teeth should be reimplanted immediately by the first capable person. If immediate reimplantation is not possible, the tooth should be stored in physiologic saline and if that is not available, the avulsed tooth should be placed in a container of milk that is packed in ice. The child's saliva is an alternative storage solution if milk is not available. The tooth should not be stored in tap water.

REFERENCES

1. Andreasen JO. The dental trauma guide. In: Andreasen JO, editor. International Association of Dental Traumatology; 2012. Avaliable at: http://www.dental traumaguide.org. Accessed October 8, 2012.
2. Jorge KO, Moyses SJ, Ferreira e Ferreira E, et al. Prevalence and factors associated to dental trauma in infants 1-3 years of age. Dent Traumatol 2009;25(2): 185–9.
3. Beltrao EM, Cavalcanti AL, Albuquerque SS, et al. Prevalence of dental trauma children aged 1-3 years in Joao Pessoa (Brazil). Eur Arch Paediatr Dent 2007; 8(3):141–3.
4. Forsberg CM, Tedestam G. Traumatic injuries to teeth in Swedish children living in an urban area. Swed Dent J 1990;14(3):115–22.
5. Baccetti T, Antonini A. Dentofacial characteristics associated with trauma to maxillary incisors in the mixed dentition. J Clin Pediatr Dent 1998;22(4):281–4.
6. Jarvinen S. Incisal overjet and traumatic injuries to upper permanent incisors. A retrospective study. Acta Odontol Scand 1978;36(6):359–62.
7. da Fonseca MA, Feigal RJ, ten Bensel RW. Dental aspects of 1248 cases of child maltreatment on file at a major county hospital. Pediatr Dent 1992;14:152–7.
8. The management of minor closed head injury in children. Committee on Quality Improvement, American Academy of Pediatrics. Commission on Clinical Policies and Research, American Academy of Family Physicians. Pediatrics 1999;104(6): 1407–15.
9. Diangelis AJ, Andreasen JO, Ebeleseder KA, et al. International Association of Dental Traumatology guidelines for the management of traumatic dental injuries: 1. Fractures and luxations of permanent teeth. Dent Traumatol 2012;28(1):2–12.
10. Holan G, Fuks AB. The diagnostic value of coronal dark-gray discoloration in primary teeth following traumatic injuries. Pediatr Dent 1996;18(3):224–7.
11. Andreasen JO, Farik B, Munksgaard EC. Long-term calcium hydroxide as a root canal dressing may increase risk of root fracture. Dent Traumatol 2002;18(3):134–7.
12. Malmgren B, Andreasen JO, Flores MT, et al. International Association of Dental Traumatology guidelines for the management of traumatic dental injuries: 3. Injuries in the primary dentition. Dent Traumatol 2012;28(3):174–82.
13. Waggoner W. Restorative dentistry for the primary dentition. In: Pinkham J, Casamassimo P, Fields H, McTigue D, Nowak A, editors. Pediatric Dentistry Infancy through Adolesence. St. Louis: Elsevier Saunders; 2005. p. 366–70.

14. Andersson L, Andreasen JO, Day P, et al. International Association of Dental Traumatology guidelines for the management of traumatic dental injuries: 2. Avulsion of permanent teeth. Dent Traumatol 2012;28(2):88–96.
15. Capp CI, Roda MI, Tamaki R, et al. Reattachment of rehydrated dental fragment using two techniques. Dent Traumatol 2009;25(1):95–9.
16. Cvek M. A clinical report on partial pulpotomy and capping with calcium hydroxide in permanent incisors with complicated crown fracture. J Endod 1978;4(8):232–7.
17. Shabahang S, Torabinejad M. Treatment of teeth with open apices using mineral trioxide aggregate. Pract Periodontics Aesthet Dent 2000;12(3):315–20 [quiz: 22].
18. Rafter M. Apexification: a review. Dent Traumatol 2005;21(1):1–8.
19. Hargreaves KM, Geisler T, Henry M, et al. Regeneration potential of the young permanent tooth: what does the future hold? Pediatr Dent 2008;30(3):253–60.
20. Thibodeau B, Trope M. Pulp revascularization of a necrotic infected immature permanent tooth: case report and review of the literature. Pediatr Dent 2007; 29(1):47–50.
21. Garcia-Godoy F, Murray PE. Recommendations for using regenerative endodontic procedures in permanent immature traumatized teeth. Dent Traumatol 2011;28(1):33–41.

Vital Pulp Therapy

Nestor Cohenca, DDS[a,b,]*, Avina Paranjpe, BDS, MS, MSD, PhD[a],
Joel Berg, DDS, MS[b]

KEYWORDS

- Vital pulp therapy • Primary teeth • Permanent teeth • Pulp • MTA

KEY POINTS

- Vital pulp therapy for children is simple.
- Vital pulp therapy is effective as long as proper assessment of the situation is made.
- Treatment is performed in the appropriate fashion with strict adherence to the proper technique.

INTRODUCTION

Vital pulp therapy is performed to preserve the health status of the tooth and its ultimate position in the arch for the expected life of the tooth. In cases of a primary tooth, the length of time for expected life is measured against the expected life of the tooth in the mouth without pulp disease or pulp therapy. Cases of permanent tooth mean long-term preservation of the tooth in a healthy state in the mouth. This article reviews the rudiments of pulp therapy for children. It is recommended that practitioners gather additional information in each of the referenced areas before engaging in pulp therapy for children. Although not specifically discussed, effective local anesthesia and rubber dam usage are always required.

The first part of this article provides insight into the basic biology of the dental pulp, the mechanisms involved in inflammation, and the reactions of the pulp to various dental materials at the cellular and molecular level whereas the second part deals with the clinical aspects of treatment of the primary and permanent dentition.

THE DENTAL PULP

The tooth pulp is a unique organ and is encased in a protective layer of dentin, which is encased by a layer of the enamel. Embryologically, histologically, and functionally, the

[a] Department of Endodontics, School of Dentistry, University of Washington, Seattle, WA, USA;
[b] Department of Pediatric Dentistry, School of Dentistry, University of Washington, Seattle, WA, USA
* Corresponding author. Department of Endodontics, School of Dentistry, University of Washington, Box 357448, Seattle, WA 98195-7448, USA.
E-mail address: cohenca@u.washington.edu

Dent Clin N Am 57 (2013) 59–73
http://dx.doi.org/10.1016/j.cden.2012.09.004
0011-8532/13/$ – see front matter © 2013 Elsevier Inc. All rights reserved.

dental.theclinics.com

dentin and the pulp are the same and are considered together, which is why they are also referred to as the pulp-dentin complex.

Zones of the Pulp

The structure of the dental pulp is similar to the other connective tissues in the body. The mature pulp demonstrates 4 morphologic zones, including

1. Odontoblastic layer: the outermost stratum of cells in a healthy pulp. It is subadjacent to the predentin and is composed of cell bodies of the odontoblasts, capillaries, nerve fibers, and dendritic cells. It is a highly specialized layer for the synthesis and secretion of the organic components of the dentin and has an epithelial layer that serves as a liner for the dental pulp.
2. Cell poor zone: also called the cell free zone of Weil because it is relatively free of cells. It is subadjacent to the odontoblastic layer and is traversed by capillaries, unmyelinated nerve fibers, and cytoplasmic processes of fibroblasts.
3. Cell-rich zone: lies subadjacent to the cell-poor zone. It has a higher number of fibroblasts with more in the central region of the pulp. The cellular components of this layer include mainly macrophages and lymphocytes. Irreversibly injured odontoblasts are replaced by cells that migrate from this layer.
4. Pulp proper: the central mass of the pulp, which consists of larger blood vessels and nerves. The connective tissue in this zone contains collagen fibers and ground substance.

Cells of the Pulp

The pulp contains numerous cells types, which include odontoblasts, fibroblasts, macrophages, dendritic cells, lymphocytes, mast cells, and undifferentiated mesenchymal stem cells. The odontoblasts are particularly important because they are responsible for dentinogenesis both during tooth development and in the mature tooth. Odontoblasts synthesize mainly type 1 collagen,[1,2] type V collagen, proteoglycans,[3] dentin sialoprotein,[4,5] and alkaline phosphatase.[4,6] The odontoblasts have odontoblastic processes that extend into the dentinal tubules and occupy most of the space of the dentinal tubules. Some studies have shown that the processes are limited to the inner third of the dentin[7,8] and other studies have demonstrate the processes extending to the dentinoenamel junction.[9,10]

Differences in the Pulp Related to Age

Aged dental pulps have various characteristics, which include the following:

1. Reduction of pulp chamber size
2. Fibrosis
3. Atrophy
4. Loss of cellularity
5. Dystrophic calcifications
6. Decreased number of stem cells
7. Degeneration of odontoblasts[11,12]

At the molecular level, one study has shown a decreased expression of connexin 43 and osteocalcin in the aged human pulp, which in turn relates to the decreased viability of the odontoblasts and the pulp cells.[13,14] Another study, by Matsuzaka and colleagues,[15] demonstrated that expression of core binding factor alpha-1 subunit and dentin sialoprotein was higher in the younger pulp whereas the adult pulp demonstrated higher levels of vascular endothelial growth factor and heat shock protein 27. The investigators concluded that the defense system in younger pulps was accomplished by calcification and in adult pulp is performed by self-defense proteins and regeneration of vessels. In terms of bacterial penetration, Kakoli and colleagues[16] showed that bacterial infection of the dentinal tubules occurs to a lesser extent in older patients than in younger patients.

PULPAL REACTIONS TO CARIES

The main functions of the pulp include (1) formation of dentin and (2) nutrition to the dentin, which is avascular, protective, and reparative.

The pulp is encased within the dentin. This provides the pulp a low-compliance environment and receives its blood supply from the blood vessels that traverse through the apical foramen. Some studies have reported that the pulp has some physiologic feedback mechanisms to counteract inflammation and increased tissue pressure, which in turn explains why inflammation of the pulp could be long standing and could heal if appropriate measures are taken in a timely manner.[17]

One of the main causes of inflammation of the pulp is dental caries. Dental caries is a progressive infection of the dentin, which may lead to inflammation and ultimately necrosis of the pulp. Caries first comes into contact with the odontoblasts. These cells are important in the defense mechanism of the pulp and have been studied extensively over the past decade. There is evidence to show that odontoblasts play an active role in innate immunity. Odontoblasts are considered highly specialized cells that have been shown to express Toll-like receptors (TLRs). TLR-2 and TLR-4 have been immune-localized in human odontoblasts.[18–20] Inflammation is a tightly regulated process and its main function is to eliminate pathogens and remove damaged tissue with the aim of restoring tissue homeostasis.[21] If the caries does progress to the pulp, it leads to inflammation, which is caused by several proinflammatory cytokines, such as interleukin (IL)-1β and tumor necrosis factor α, and chemokines, which cause cell death, increased vascular permeability, and an increase in inflammatory cells into the area along with production of acute phase proteins.[22,23] Removal of caries may cause cessation of the inflammation but there is a continuous production of these proinflammatory cytokines, which could lead to irreversible pulpal damage followed by necrosis.[24]

PULPAL REACTIONS TO DENTAL MATERIALS

Once a tooth is affected by caries, some form of intervention is necessary to prevent further inflammation and ultimately necrosis. Caries excavation followed by placement of a restoration is necessary. Hence, this discussion has 2 parts: first, the materials that are placed in direct contact with the pulp, and second, restorative materials placed in the tooth after excavation of caries.

Reactions of the Pulp to Materials Used During Pulp Capping or Pulpotomy Procedures

Pulpotomy and pulp capping are indicated for teeth that have had a pulp exposure after trauma or injury, which may include the process of caries excavation in developing or mature teeth. These procedures offer good alternatives to root canal therapy for teeth with immature or mature apices when pulp is exposed with reversible injury and without signs of inflammation, offering a more conservative approach. Ultimately, the goal of treating the exposed pulp with an appropriate pulp capping material is to promote the dentinogenic potential of the pulpal cells.[25] Historically many different materials have been used for these procedures, including resin-modified glass ionomer cements, tricalcium phosphates, hydrophilic resins, and calcium hydroxide. The success of different pulp capping materials has been measured by thickness of the dentinal bridge, morphology of the dentinal bridge, intensity of pulpal inflammation, presence of odontoblasts cells, and biocompatibility.[26]

Historically, the material used during pulp capping procedures has been calcium hydroxide. Calcium hydroxide has been considered the gold standard for pulp capping; however, previous research has shown that it is not ideally suited for this procedure. The opponents of calcium hydroxide for direct pulp capping procedures cite 3 major causes of failure:

1. The porosity of the dentinal bridge that is produced
2. Calcium hydroxide adhering poorly to dentin
3. Inability to provide a long-term seal against microleakage[26,27]

The porosity of this dentinal bridge potentially allows recolonization of bacteria, thereby leading to failure of pulp capping procedures.[27] Other studies have reported that calcium hydroxide caused a layer of necrosis of the pulp tissue when used in pulp capping procedures.[28]

Another pulp capping material recently developed is mineral trioxide aggregate (MTA). This material has drawn much interest due to its many applications. MTA has demonstrated significantly greater frequency of dentin bridge formation, thicker and less porous dentin, and less pulp inflammation compared with calcium hydroxide.[26,29–31] Recent research has shown that MTA, when placed in direct contact with the human dental pulp cells, differentiated them into odontoblast-like cells.[32]

No layer of necrosis was seen in the pulp when MTA was used for pulp capping.[28] At the cellular level, MTA has also been shown to induce the recruitment and proliferation of undifferentiated cells to form a dentinal bridge, while reducing inflammation compared with calcium hydroxide.[26] Another study showed that MTA causes neutrophils to be recruited to the site of injury, which is important in the process of inflammation.[33] Nair and colleagues[34] also demonstrated decreased inflammation when MTA was used compared with calcium hydroxide. On the molecular level, MTA has been shown to induce the secretion of angiogenic factors, such as vascular endothelial growth factor, which plays an important role in healing.[6,32] Other studies have shown that MTA induced cells to secrete IL-8 and IL-1β. IL-1β has been shown to induce the synthesis of collagen, resulting in a more organized response of the pulp and assisting in the healing process.[35–37] Other studies in animal models have shown that MTA down-regulated inflammatory cytokines, such as interferon-gamma, CCL5 (also referred to as regulated on activation, normal T-cell expressed, and secreted [RANTES]), and IL-1α,[38] and suppressed the proliferation of some microorganisms and inhibited the production of certain T_H1 and T_H2 cytokines.[39]

Recently a new material has been introduced, BioAggregate (BA) (Innovative Bio-Ceramix, Vancouver, British Columbia, Canada). BA is white nanoparticle ceramic cement with many different applications, like MTA.[40] Studies have reported this material to have similar cytotoxicity levels as MTA[41,42] De-Deus and colleagues[43] found that BA was as biocompatible as MTA and another study reported that BA up-regulated the gene expression of collagen 1, osteocalcin, and osteopontin in osteoblasts and differentiation of human periodontal ligament fibroblasts compared with MTA.[44,45] BA has also been shown have antifungal and antibacterial activity.[46,47] Similar to MTA, this material induced secretion of IL-1β, IL-6, and IL-8.[48] Further research with the new material, however, is ongoing.

Pulpal Reactions to Composite-Based Restorative Materials

Some of the more common restorative materials currently used are resin based. Although the use of these materials is aesthetically appealing in patients, they carry the risk of local and systemic adverse effects. The potential risks are direct damage to the cells (cytotoxicity) and induction of immune-based hypersensitivity reactions.[49] Resin monomers, such as 2-hydroxyethyl methacrylate (HEMA) and triethyleneglycol dimethacrylate (TEGDMA), are shown to influence the differentiation of human pulp cells into odontoblasts.[50] Studies have previously shown that HEMA induces apoptosis in different cell types[49] and also in dental pulp stem cells and in odontoblast-like cells. HEMA-induced apoptosis has been linked to the decrease in intracellular glutathione levels and the production of reactive oxygen species in the cells.[51–55] At the molecular level, HEMA and TEGDMA have shown to cause cell death/apoptosis in the pulp cells by a decrease in important transcription factors, such as nuclear factor κB (NF-κB) and increase in c-Jun N-terminal kinases (JNK).[56] NF-κB is the major transcription factor that is involved in the regulation of a variety of genes responsible for survival of the cells.[57,58] The activity of NF-κB is tightly regulated by cytokines and other external regulators.[59,60] JNK belongs to the family of mitogen-activated protein kinases that comprise of a group of serine/threonine kinases, which are responsible for phosphorylation and mediation of signal transduction from extracellular stimuli. It is believed that activation of JNK inhibits cell growth and induces cell death.[61–64] Other studies have demonstrated that HEMA causes increased phophorylation of extracellular-signal-regulated kinases (ERK 1 and 2) and decreased phosphorylation of phosphokinase B (p-AKT).[65,66] The full spectrum of signals responsible for the induction apoptosis in the cells by HEMA and TEGDMA is not established yet, but it involves several different pathways. A better insight into mechanisms of toxicity of dental materials is important for understanding the potential of these materials to cause adverse health effects in a clinical setting.

Knowing the background about the dental pulp, the various cell types, and their interactions with each other and with various dental materials is important because this could ultimately lead to a better treatment modalities. Hence, the second part of this review deals with the clinical aspects of treatment of the primary and permanent dentition.

PRIMARY DENTITION
Anterior

When decay or tooth preparation extends into the pulp chamber of the primary incisor or canine, first, an assessment of the vitality of the pulp must be made. This should be done before the procedure via radiographic assessment or by direct examination of pulp and its color, texture, and bleeding during the procedure. If the pulp does not bleed at all or bleeds at a hemorrhagic level, it may be infected beyond the coronal pulp, and a pulpectomy may be in order. In this instance, the coronal and radicular pulps should be removed all the way to the apex of the tooth. The radicular pulp chamber may be filled with a resorbable paste of either zinc oxide–eugenol or, preferably, calcium hydroxide with iodoform within the paste. The paste is condensed into the radicular pulp chamber after careful pulp extirpation, cleaning of the canal, and irrigation with saline. Generally, sodium hypochlorite has not been used to clean the pulp canals of primary teeth. The coronal chamber should be filled with glass ionomer or resin-modified glass ionomer. The crown is then restored with a stainless steel crown, a composite strip crown, or a preveneered, commercially available composite-faced stainless steel crown. If there are signs of early external root resorption, radiolucency beyond the confines of the pulp chamber related to the tooth or other signs of disease, or inadequate tooth structure to support a restoration, the tooth may need to be extracted.

Molars

When decay or tooth preparation extends into the coronal pulp, and the pulp is deemed vital (as described previously), a pulpotomy may be performed. The entire coronal pulp is removed circumferentially with a large round bur, pulling coronally to adequately deroof the pulp chamber and to avoid leaving any ledges or pulp tissue therein. The radicular orifices are assessed to determine that bleeding can be controlled only by direct pressure with a damp cotton piece for a minute or 2. There is some debate as to whether the remaining radicular pulp orifices should be further treated with a medicament, such as formocresol or ferric sulfate. The literature and standard of care is to use one of these agents (not discussed in this article because of the length limitations); however, there seems to be a directional change toward sealing the orifices completely as the primary objective. It is likely that recommendations going forward will require sealing the orifices as the main objective. The best sealing agents seem to be MTA or glass ionomer. Therefore, after achieving hemostasis on the radicular pulp orifices, and after using a medicament (if desired), the orifices must be sealed with one of these agents. A material that further seals, such as glass ionomer or resin-modified glass ionomer, should then be used to fill the coronal pulp chamber. A stainless steel crown is the restoration of choice after performing a primary molar pulpotomy. If the pulp tissue is nonvital or the bleeding cannot be controlled at the level of the orifice, a pulpectomy should be performed. Canals should be cleaned carefully but not significantly instrumented (primary roots are narrow and curved and there is a risk of perforation or extension beyond the apex). Canals and the pulp chamber should be filled (as described previously) for primary anterior teeth. A stainless steel crown is then used to restore the tooth. As with a primary anterior tooth, when there is disease beyond the confines of the tooth related to the tooth, consideration for extraction must be given. The tooth itself, however, is the best space maintainer, and space loss in the primary molar area is a significant long-term issue for patients. If there is the ability to retain the tooth in the mouth via pulpectomy and careful monitoring of the tooth to reduce or eliminate local infection, while waiting for a permanent molar to erupt (in the case of second primary molar infection), this treatment option may be performed with careful monitoring as a transitional treatment. In addition to maintaining the tooth, this option will ease and make a band and loop from permanent molar to primary first molar well tolerated (compared with the distal shoe appliance).

PERMANENT DENTITION

Endodontics is defined as the branch of dentistry concerned with the morphology, physiology, and pathology of the human dental pulp and periradicular tissues. The ultimate endodontics goal could be defined, however, as the prevention and/or elimination of apical periodontitis. The cause of apical periodontitis is toxic metabolites and byproducts released from microorganisms within the canal and diffused into periapical tissues, eliciting inflammatory responses and bone resorption. Thus, in clinical terms, a necrotic infected pulp is required for apical periodontitis to be present. Conversely, if the pulp is vital, there should be few or no bacteria present in the root pulp space and thus the disease (apical periodontitis) should not be present.

Therefore, preservation and treatment of the vital pulp are critical for the prevention of apical periodontitis.

VITAL PULP THERAPY IN PERMANENT TEETH

Vital pulp therapy has a high success rate if the following conditions are met: (1) the pulp is not inflamed, (2) hemorrhage is properly controlled, (3) a nontoxic capping material is applied, and (4) the capping material and restoration seal out bacteria.

Indirect Pulp Therapy

Indirect pulp capping has been defined as a procedure in which a small amount of carious dentin is retained in deep areas of cavity preparation to avoid an exposure of the pulp. A medicament is then placed over the carious dentin to stimulate and encourage pulp recovery.

Indications

1. Vital pulp
2. Normal radiographic findings
3. No history of spontaneous, lingering, or severe pain
4. No extensive restoration or full crown requirements

Contraindications

1. History of spontaneous pain or signs of irreversible pulpitis
2. Clinical or radiographic evidence of pulpal or periradicular pathosis
3. Carious exposure
4. Tooth requires extensive restoration or full crown

Technique

1. Remove soft leathery caries affected tooth structure until dentin consistency changes or pulp exposure is imminent.
2. Disinfect the cavity using 2.5% sodium hypochlorite for at least 1 minute.
3. Place calcium hydroxide or glass ionomer directly over the carious region.
4. Place a permanent restoration.

In a retrospective study, Gruythuysen and colleagues[67] examined clinically and radiographically the 3-year survival of teeth treated with indirect pulp therapy performed between 2000 and 2004. After placement of a layer of resin-modified glass ionomer as liner over carious dentin, the teeth were restored. Failure was defined as the presence of either a clinical symptom (pain, swelling, or fistula) or radiologic abnormality at recall. The survival rate was 96% for primary molars (mean survival time, 146 weeks) and 93% for permanent teeth (mean survival time, 178 weeks). This study shows that indirect pulp therapy performed in primary and permanent teeth of young patients may result in a high 3-year survival rate. Other studies had given a lower prognosis to indirect pulp therapy, however, especially in permanent teeth. With the development of more biocompatible materials with high sealing properties, these teeth might have a better outcome with direct pulp therapy.

Direct Pulp Therapy

Direct pulp capping is defined as the placement of a medicament on a pulp that has been exposed in the course of excavating the last portions of deep dental caries. The rationale behind this treatment is the encouragement of young healthy pulps to initiate a dentin bridge and wall off the exposure site. A good rule of thumb limits the diameter of the exposure site to less than 1.5 mm.

Indications

1. Mechanically or traumatically exposed primary and young permanent teeth
2. No history of spontaneous or irreversible inflamed pulp
3. Vital pulp
4. Normal radiographic findings
5. Controlled hemorrhage
6. Limited restorative treatment

Contraindications

1. Spontaneous pain
2. Large carious exposures
3. Radiographic evidence of pulpal or periradicular pathosis
4. Calcifications in the pulp chamber
5. Excessive hemorrhage encountered
6. Exposures with purulent or serous exudates

Technique

1. Remove all peripheral caries before removing the deepest caries.
2. Control the hemorrhage with a sterile cotton pellet moistened with sterile saline.
3. Disinfect the cavity using 2.5% sodium hypochlorite for at least 1 minute.
4. Place calcium hydroxide, MTAs, or BA directly over the exposure site; do not force it into the pulp.
5. Cover the capping material with glass ionomer and restore permanently.

As discussed previously, there are various materials that have been tried and tested for pulp capping procedures. When considering the capping material, current evidence in the literature has consistently demonstrated a better outcome when using MTA. Aeinehchi and colleagues[68] compared the use of MTA and calcium hydroxide in direct pulp capping cases using 11 pairs of third molars (patients 20–25 years old) with pulps mechanically exposed and capped with either MTA or calcium hydroxide, covered with zinc oxide–eugenol, and restored with amalgam. Teeth were extracted and then histologically evaluated at 1 week and 2, 3, 4, and 6 months. Odontoblastic layers appeared earlier; less hyperemia, inflammation, and necrosis were noted; and dentinal bridges were more pronounced in the MTA-treated teeth. In a different randomized clinical study, Nair and colleagues investigated the pulpal response to direct pulp capping in healthy human teeth with MTA versus calcium hydroxide cement (Dycal) as control. MTA was clinically easier to use as a direct pulp capping agent and resulted in less pulpal inflammation and more predictable hard tissue barrier formation than Dycal. Therefore, MTA or equivalent products should be the material of choice for direct pulp capping procedures instead of hard-setting calcium hydroxide cements.

From a clinical perspective, the control of the hemorrhage is critical to determine the level of pulp inflammation. In cases of persistent bleeding, partial pulpotomy might be indicated.

Partial Pulpotomy

According to the American Association of Endodontists glossary, partial pulpotomy is defined as the removal of a small portion of the vital coronal pulp as a means of preserving the remaining coronal and radicular pulp tissues[69] to encourage continued physiologic development and formation of the root end. In children and young adults, teeth with traumatic pulp exposure can be treated successfully (96%) with partial pulpotomy and calcium hydroxide.[70] The procedure is also known as Cvek pulpotomy. Cvek and colleagues[71] investigated the depth of inflammatory reactions of adult monkey pulps exposed by fracture or cavity prep at different time intervals and found that inflammation extended 1.5 mm to 2 mm into the pulp at the 48-hour mark and only 0.8 mm to 2.2 mm after 1 week. Thus, to be effective, calcium hydroxide needs to be in contact with noninflamed tissue located approximately 2 mm of pulp beneath exposure site. In 1987, Fuks and colleagues[72] performed partial pulpotomy on 63 teeth with different types and severity of traumatic injuries and demonstrated a 94% success rate. No correlations were found between healing and size of pulp exposure, type of trauma, time frame, and root development.

Indications

1. Carious or traumatically exposed primary and permanent teeth
2. Vital pulp, which responds to sensitivity tests
3. Normal radiographic findings
4. Controlled hemorrhage
5. Limited to moderate restorative treatment

Contraindications

1. Spontaneous pain
2. Radiographic evidence of pulpal or periradicular pathosis
3. Calcifications in the pulp chamber
4. Excessive hemorrhage encountered
5. Exposures with purulent or serous exudates

Technique

1. Access the tooth using a high-speed bur.
2. Using a sterile round bur and/or a sharp spoon, amputate the coronal pulp.
3. Clean canal walls with moistened sterile cotton pellet.
4. Apply pressure with a moist sterile cotton pellet on the pulp stump to control hemorrhage.
5. Disinfect the pulp wound and cavity with 2% chlorhexidine gluconate.
6. MTA, BA, or calcium hydroxide is laid over the pulp stump to a thickness of 2–3 mm.

Vital Pulp Therapy on Immature Teeth

For cases of open apexes, maintaining the pulp vital is essential for the development of the root and maturation of the whole tooth. According to the American Association of Endodontists glossary, apexogenesis is defined as a vital pulp therapy procedure performed to encourage continued physiologic development and formation of the root end. The term is frequently used to describe therapy performed to encourage the continuation of this process. The term, *maturogenesis*, was recently introduced by Weisleder and Benitez[73] and defined as physiologic root development not restricted to the apical segment. The continued deposition of dentin occurs throughout the length of the root, providing greater strength and resistance to fracture. Patel and Cohenca[74] also presented a case that demonstrates the use of MTA as a direct pulp capping material for the purpose of continued maturogenesis of the root. Clinical and radiographic follow-up demonstrated a vital pulp and physiologic root development in comparison with the contralateral tooth. MTA can be considered as an effective material for vital pulp therapy, with the goal of maturogenesis.

Treatment of Nonvital Immature Teeth

Apexification is defined as a method of inducing a calcified barrier in a root with an open apex or the continued apical development of an incompletely formed root in teeth with necrotic pulp.

CLASSIC TECHNIQUE USING CALCIUM HYDROXIDE

1. Remove necrotic pulpal tissue to a level 1-mm short of the apical foramen. The use of negative pressure irrigation is highly recommended for safe and proper disinfection.
2. Fill root canal with calcium hydroxide and seal the access.
3. Recall every 6 months until evidence of an apical barrier. This process can take anywhere between 6 to 24 months.
4. Verify barrier formation clinically before obturation with gutta-percha.

Felippe and colleagues[75] evaluated the influence of renewing calcium hydroxide paste on apexification and periapical healing of teeth in dogs with incomplete root formation and previously contaminated canals. Replacement of calcium hydroxide paste was not necessary for apexification to occur; however, replacement of calcium hydroxide paste significantly reduced the intensity of the inflammatory process. In young immature teeth with undeveloped roots and nonvital pulp, the conventional treatment (apexification) can take up to 18 months. Such long treatment planning may cause crown-root fracture at the cervical area (thin and weak dentinal walls), coronal leakage and recontamination of the root canal space and dentinal tubules, lack of compliance from the patients to come to several appointments, and failure to provide an esthetic and final restoration of the crown.

ALTERNATIVE TECHNIQUE USING MTA

Apexification procedures should be completed immediately after the infection control is achieved, allowing strengthening the cervical third and providing an immediate permanent and esthetic restoration. In 2001, the use of MTA was suggested as a replacement of long-term apexification with calcium hydroxide.[76] Several procedures and materials have been used to induce root-end barrier formation. In 2001, Witherspoon and Ham[76] reported promising results when using MTA in 1-visit apexification treatment of immature teeth with necrotic pulps. Moreover, the use of an intracanal medication is not necessary when using MTA as an apical plug. Overall, the development of clinical applications of MTA has increased significantly the treatment outcome of vital and nonvital therapy.

REGENERATIVE ENDODONTICS

The process of apexification entails formation of calcified barrier for a tooth with an open apex. However, even if rendered successful, apexification procedures will leave a short root with thin dentinal walls with a high risk of root fracture.[77] Root fractures commonly occur in the cervical third, and have been shown to have a rate of about 28-77% depending on the stage of root development.[78]

Regenerative endodontic procedures have been previously described as biologically based procedures designed to replace damaged structures, including dentin and root structures, as well as cells of the pulp-dentin complex.[79] Recently, pulp revascularization procedures for the treatment of immature teeth with necrotic pulps and apical periodontitis have gained much attention as a result of encouraging results seen from numerous in vitro and in vivo studies.[80,81] The advantage of revascularization procedures over apexification procedures is that it allows continued maturation of the root.[82]

The procedure is indicated only for immature teeth presenting with pulp necrosis and apical periodontitis and involves disinfection of the canal and induction of intracanal bleeding,[83] which introduces stem cells originated at the apical papilla (SCAP).[84] SCAP are a recently discovered and isolated population of mesenchymal stem cells (MSCs) residing in the apical papilla of incompletely developed teeth.[84] SCAP are thought to be derived from the dental papilla and help form primary dentin to aid in root development.[85] Mineral Trioxide Aggregate (MTA) is then placed over the blood clot and the crown restored. The process of revascularization is innovative in that it could in the future, replace treatments such as apexification as some reports have shown it to provide a better outcome.[86,87]

SUMMARY

Vital pulp therapy for children is simple and effective as long as the proper assessment of the situation is made and treatment is performed in the appropriate fashion with strict adherence to the proper technique.

REFERENCES

1. Lesot H, Osman M, Ruch JV. Immunofluorescent localization of collagens, fibronectin, and laminin during terminal differentiation of odontoblasts. Dev Biol 1981; 82:371–81.
2. Orsini G, Ruggeri A Jr, Mazzoni A, et al. Immunohistochemical identification of type I and type III collagen and chondroitin sulphate in human pre-dentine: a correlative FEI-SEM/TEM study. Int Endod J 2007;40:669–78.
3. Goldberg M, Takagi M. Dentine proteoglycans: composition, ultrastructure and functions. Histochem J 1993;25:781–806.
4. Butler WT, D'Souza RN, Bronckers AL, et al. Recent investigations on dentin specific proteins. Proc Finn Dent Soc 1992;88(Suppl 1):369–76.
5. Butler WT, Bhown M, Brunn JC, et al. Isolation, characterization and immunolocalization of a 53-kDal dentin sialoprotein (DSP). Matrix 1992;12:343–51.
6. Paranjpe A, Cacalano NA, Hume WR, et al. N-acetylcysteine protects dental pulp stromal cells from HEMA-induced apoptosis by inducing differentiation of the cells. Free Radic Biol Med 2007;43:1394–408.
7. Byers MR, Sugaya A. Odontoblast processes in dentin revealed by fluorescent Di-I. J Histochem Cytochem 1995;43:159–68.
8. Thomas HF. The extent of the odontoblast process in human dentin. J Dent Res 1979;58:2207–18.
9. Sigal MJ, Pitaru S, Aubin JE, et al. A combined scanning electron microscopy and immunofluorescence study demonstrating that the odontoblast process extends to the dentinoenamel junction in human teeth. Anat Rec 1984;210:453–62.
10. Sigal MJ, Aubin JE, Ten Cate AR, et al. The odontoblast process extends to the dentinoenamel junction: an immunocytochemical study of rat dentine. J Histochem Cytochem 1984;32:872–7.
11. Bernick S, Nedelman C. Effect of aging on the human pulp. J Endod 1975;1:88–94.

12. Ketterl W. Age-induced changes in the teeth and their attachment apparatus. Int Dent J 1983;33:262–71.
13. Muramatsu T, Hamano H, Ogami K, et al. Reduction of connexin 43 expression in aged human dental pulp. Int Endod J 2004;37:814–8.
14. Muramatsu T, Hamano H, Ogami K, et al. Reduction of osteocalcin expression in aged human dental pulp. Int Endod J 2005;38:817–21.
15. Matsuzaka K, Muramatsu T, Katakura A, et al. Changes in the homeostatic mechanism of dental pulp with age: expression of the core-binding factor alpha-1, dentin sialoprotein, vascular endothelial growth factor, and heat shock protein 27 messenger RNAs. J Endod 2008;34:818–21.
16. Kakoli P, Nandakumar R, Romberg E, et al. The effect of age on bacterial penetration of radicular dentin. J Endod 2009;35:78–81.
17. Heyeraas KJ, Berggreen E. Interstitial fluid pressure in normal and inflamed pulp. Crit Rev Oral Biol Med 1999;10:328–36.
18. Veerayutthwilai O, Byers MR, Pham TT, et al. Differential regulation of immune responses by odontoblasts. Oral Microbiol Immunol 2007;22:5–13.
19. Jiang HW, Zhang W, Ren BP, et al. Expression of toll like receptor 4 in normal human odontoblasts and dental pulp tissue. J Endod 2006;32:747–51.
20. Mutoh N, Tani-Ishii N, Tsukinoki K, et al. Expression of toll-like receptor 2 and 4 in dental pulp. J Endod 2007;33:1183–6.
21. Soehnlein O, Lindbom L. Phagocyte partnership during the onset and resolution of inflammation. Nat Rev Immunol 2010;10:427–39.
22. Farges JC, Carrouel F, Keller JF, et al. Cytokine production by human odontoblast-like cells upon Toll-like receptor-2 engagement. Immunobiology 2011;216:513–7.
23. Min KS, Kwon YY, Lee HJ, et al. Effects of proinflammatory cytokines on the expression of mineralization markers and heme oxygenase-1 in human pulp cells. J Endod 2006;32:39–43.
24. Takeuchi O, Akira S. Pattern recognition receptors and inflammation. Cell 2010; 140:805–20.
25. Schroder U. Effects of calcium hydroxide-containing pulp-capping agents on pulp cell migration, proliferation, and differentiation. J Dent Res 1985;64(Spec No): 541–8.
26. Holland R, Filho JA, de Souza V, et al. Mineral trioxide aggregate repair of lateral root perforations. J Endod 2001;27:281–4.
27. Faraco IM Jr, Holland R. Response of the pulp of dogs to capping with mineral trioxide aggregate or a calcium hydroxide cement. Dent Traumatol 2001;17: 163–6.
28. Dammaschke T, Wolff P, Sagheri D, et al. Mineral trioxide aggregate for direct pulp capping: a histologic comparison with calcium hydroxide in rat molars. Quintessence Int 2010;41:e20–30.
29. Nair PN, Duncan HF, Pitt Ford TR, et al. Histological, ultrastructural and quantitative investigations on the response of healthy human pulps to experimental capping with Mineral Trioxide Aggregate: a randomized controlled trial. 2008. Int Endod J 2009;42:422–44.
30. Ford TR, Torabinejad M, McKendry DJ, et al. Use of mineral trioxide aggregate for repair of furcal perforations. Oral Surg Oral Med Oral Pathol Oral Radiol Endod 1995;79:756–63.
31. Ford TR, Torabinejad M, Abedi HR, et al. Using mineral trioxide aggregate as a pulp-capping material. J Am Dent Assoc 1996;127:1491–4.

32. Paranjpe A, Zhang H, Johnson JD. Effects of mineral trioxide aggregate on human dental pulp cells after pulp-capping procedures. J Endod 2010;36:1042–7.
33. Gomes AC, Filho JE, de Oliveira SH. MTA-induced neutrophil recruitment: a mechanism dependent on IL-1beta, MIP-2, and LTB4. Oral Surg Oral Med Oral Pathol Oral Radiol Endod 2008;106:450–6.
34. Nair PN, Duncan HF, Pitt Ford TR, et al. Histological, ultrastructural and quantitative investigations on the response of healthy human pulps to experimental capping with mineral trioxide aggregate: a randomized controlled trial. Int Endod J 2008;41:128–50.
35. Barkhordar RA, Ghani QP, Russell TR, et al. Interleukin-1beta activity and collagen synthesis in human dental pulp fibroblasts. J Endod 2002;28:157–9.
36. Cavalcanti BN, Rode Sde M, Franca CM, et al. Pulp capping materials exert an effect on the secretion of IL-1beta and IL-8 by migrating human neutrophils. Braz Oral Res 2011;25:13–8.
37. Ferreira DC, Brito DG, Cavalcanti BN. Cytokine production from human primary teeth pulp fibroblasts stimulated by different pulpotomy agents. J Dent Child (Chic) 2009;76:194–8.
38. Barbosa Silva MJ, Vieira LQ, Sobrinho AP. The effects of mineral trioxide aggregates on cytokine production by mouse pulp tissue. Oral Surg Oral Med Oral Pathol Oral Radiol Endod 2008;105:e70–6.
39. Rezende TM, Vieira LQ, Sobrinho AP, et al. The influence of mineral trioxide aggregate on adaptive immune responses to endodontic pathogens in mice. J Endod 2008;34:1066–71.
40. Zhang H, Pappen FG, Haapasalo M. Dentin enhances the antibacterial effect of mineral trioxide aggregate and bioaggregate. J Endod 2009;35:221–4.
41. Damas BA, Wheater MA, Bringas JS, et al. Cytotoxicity comparison of mineral trioxide aggregates and EndoSequence bioceramic root repair materials. J Endod 2011;37:372–5.
42. Alanezi AZ, Jiang J, Safavi KE, et al. Cytotoxicity evaluation of endosequence root repair material. Oral Surg Oral Med Oral Pathol Oral Radiol Endod 2010; 109:e122–5.
43. De-Deus G, Canabarro A, Alves G, et al. Optimal cytocompatibility of a bioceramic nanoparticulate cement in primary human mesenchymal cells. J Endod 2009;35:1387–90.
44. Yan P, Yuan Z, Jiang H, et al. Effect of bioaggregate on differentiation of human periodontal ligament fibroblasts. Int Endod J 2010;43:1116–21.
45. Yuan Z, Peng B, Jiang H, et al. Effect of bioaggregate on mineral-associated gene expression in osteoblast cells. J Endod 2010;36:1145–8.
46. Dohaithem A, Al-Nasser A, Al-Badah A, et al. An in vitro evaluation of antifungal activity of bioaggregate. Oral Surg Oral Med Oral Pathol Oral Radiol Endod 2011; 112:e27–30.
47. Lovato KF, Sedgley CM. Antibacterial activity of endosequence root repair material and proroot MTA against clinical isolates of Enterococcus faecalis. J Endod 2011;37:1542–6.
48. Ciasca M, Aminoshariae A, Jin G, et al. A comparison of the cytotoxicity and proinflammatory cytokine production of EndoSequence root repair material and ProRoot mineral trioxide aggregate in human osteoblast cell culture using reverse-transcriptase polymerase chain reaction. J Endod 2012;38:486–9.
49. Paranjpe A, Bordador LC, Wang MY, et al. Resin monomer 2-hydroxyethyl methacrylate (HEMA) is a potent inducer of apoptotic cell death in human and mouse cells. J Dent Res 2005;84:172–7.

50. About I, Camps J, Mitsiadis TA, et al. Influence of resinous monomers on the differentiation in vitro of human pulp cells into odontoblasts. J Biomed Mater Res 2002;63:418–23.
51. Stanislawski L, Daniau X, Lauti A, et al. Factors responsible for pulp cell cytotoxicity induced by resin-modified glass ionomer cements. J Biomed Mater Res 1999;48:277–88.
52. Stanislawski L, Lefeuvre M, Bourd K, et al. TEGDMA-induced toxicity in human fibroblasts is associated with early and drastic glutathione depletion with subsequent production of oxygen reactive species. J Biomed Mater Res A 2003;66: 476–82.
53. Walther UI, Walther SC, Liebl B, et al. Cytotoxicity of ingredients of various dental materials and related compounds in L2- and A549 cells. J Biomed Mater Res 2002;63:643–9.
54. Hunag TH, Lii CK, Kao CT. Root canal sealers cause cytotoxicity and oxidative damage in hepatocytes. J Biomed Mater Res 2001;54:390–5.
55. Stanislawski L, Soheili-Majd E, Perianin A, et al. Dental restorative biomaterials induce glutathione depletion in cultured human gingival fibroblast: protective effect of N-acetyl cysteine. J Biomed Mater Res 2000;51:469–74.
56. Paranjpe A, Cacalano NA, Hume WR, et al. N-acetyl cysteine mediates protection from 2-hydroxyethyl methacrylate induced apoptosis via nuclear factor kappa B-dependent and independent pathways: potential involvement of JNK. Toxicol Sci 2009;108:356–66.
57. Jewett A, Cacalano NA, Teruel A, et al. Inhibition of nuclear factor kappa B (NFkappaB) activity in oral tumor cells prevents depletion of NK cells and increases their functional activation. Cancer Immunol Immunother 2006;55: 1052–63.
58. Beg AA, Baltimore D. An essential role for NF-kappaB in preventing TNF-alpha-induced cell death. Science 1996;274:782–4.
59. Baeuerle PA, Henkel T. Function and activation of NF-kappa B in the immune system. Annu Rev Immunol 1994;12:141–79.
60. Verma IM, Stevenson JK, Schwarz EM, et al. Rel/NF-kappa B/I kappa B family: intimate tales of association and dissociation. Genes Dev 1995;9:2723–35.
61. Kyriakis JM, Banerjee P, Nikolakaki E, et al. The stress-activated protein kinase subfamily of c-Jun kinases. Nature 1994;369:156–60.
62. Xia Z, Dickens M, Raingeaud J, et al. Opposing effects of ERK and JNK-p38 MAP kinases on apoptosis. Science 1995;270:1326–31.
63. Kyriakis JM, Avruch J. Sounding the alarm: protein kinase cascades activated by stress and inflammation. J Biol Chem 1996;271:24313–6.
64. Kyriakis JM, Avruch J. Protein kinase cascades activated by stress and inflammatory cytokines. Bioessays 1996;18:567–77.
65. Samuelsen JT, Dahl JE, Karlsson S, et al. Apoptosis induced by the monomers HEMA and TEGDMA involves formation of ROS and differential activation of the MAP-kinases p38, JNK and ERK. Dent Mater 2007;23:34–9.
66. Spagnuolo G, D'Anto V, Valletta R, et al. Effect of 2-hydroxyethyl methacrylate on human pulp cell survival pathways ERK and AKT. J Endod 2008;34:684–8.
67. Gruythuysen RJ, van Strijp AJ, Wu MK. Long-term survival of indirect pulp treatment performed in primary and permanent teeth with clinically diagnosed deep carious lesions. J Endod 2010;36:1490–3.
68. Aeinehchi M, Eslami B, Ghanbariha M, et al. Mineral trioxide aggregate (MTA) and calcium hydroxide as pulp-capping agents in human teeth: a preliminary report. Int Endod J 2003;36:225–31.

69. American Association of Endodontists. Glossary of endodontic terms. American Association of Endodontists, Chicago, IL; 2012.

70. Cvek M. A clinical report on partial pulpotomy and capping with calcium hydroxide in permanent incisors with complicated crown fracture. J Endod 1978;4:232–7.

71. Cvek M, Cleaton-Jones PE, Austin JC, et al. Pulp reactions to exposure after experimental crown fractures or grinding in adult monkeys. J Endod 1982;8: 391–7.

72. Fuks AB, Cosack A, Klein H, et al. Partial pulpotomy as a treatment alternative for exposed pulps in crown-fractured permanent incisors. Endod Dent Traumatol 1987;3:100–2.

73. Weisleder R, Benitez CR. Maturogenesis: is it a new concept? J Endod 2003; 29(11):776–8.

74. Patel R, Cohenca N. Maturogenesis of a cariously exposed immature permanent tooth using MTA for direct pulp capping: a case report. Dent Traumatol 2006;22: 328–33.

75. Felippe MC, Felippe WT, Marques MM, et al. The effect of the renewal of calcium hydroxide paste on the apexification and periapical healing of teeth with incomplete root formation. Int Endod J 2005;38:436–42.

76. Witherspoon DE, Ham K. One-visit apexification: technique for inducing root-end barrier formation in apical closures. Pract Proced Aesthet Dent 2001;13:455–60.

77. Andreasen FM, Andreasen JO, Bayer T. Prognosis of root-fractured permanent incisors–prediction of healing modalities. Endod Dent Traumatol 1989;5(1):11–22.

78. Cvek M. Prognosis of luxated non-vital maxillary incisors treated with calcium hydroxide and filled with gutta-percha. A retrospective clinical study. Endod Dent Traumatol 1992;8(2):45–55.

79. Murray PE, Garcia-Godoy F, Hargreaves KM. Regenerative endodontics: a review of current status and a call for action. J Endod 2007;33(4):377–90.

80. Bose R, Nummikoski P, Hargreaves K. A retrospective evaluation of radiographic outcomes in immature teeth with necrotic root canal systems treated with regenerative endodontic procedures. J Endod 2009;35(10):1343–9.

81. Iwaya SI, Ikawa M, Kubota M. Revascularization of an immature permanent tooth with apical periodontitis and sinus tract. Dent Traumatol 2001;17(4):185–7.

82. Yamauchi N, Yamauchi S, Nagaoka H, Duggan D, Zhong S, Lee SM, et al. Tissue engineering strategies for immature teeth with apical periodontitis. J Endod 2011; 37(3):390–7.

83. Banchs F, Trope M. Revascularization of immature permanent teeth with apical periodontitis: new treatment protocol? J Endod 2004;30(4):196–200.

84. Huang GT, Sonoyama W, Liu Y, et al. The hidden treasure in apical papilla: the potential role in pulp/dentin regeneration and bioroot engineering. J Endod 2008;34(6):645–51.

85. Sonoyama W, Liu Y, Yamaza T, et al. Characterization of the apical papilla and its residing stem cells from human immature permanent teeth: a pilot study. J Endod 2008;34(2):166–71.

86. Reynolds K, Johnson JD, Cohenca N. Pulp revascularization of necrotic bilateral bicuspids using a modified novel technique to eliminate potential coronal discolouration: a case report. Int Endod J 2009;42(1):84–92.

87. Jeeruphan T, Jantarat J, Yanpiset K, et al. Mahidol study 1: comparison of radiographic and survival outcomes of immature teeth treated with either regenerative endodontic or apexification methods: a retrospective study. J Endod 2012; 38(10):1330–6. Epub 2012 Aug 15.

Restorative Dentistry for Children

Kevin J. Donly, DDS, MS

KEYWORDS

- Pediatric • Dentistry • Restorations • Resin-based composite
- Glass ionomer cement • Stainless steel crowns

KEY POINTS

- The indications and contraindications of the use of dental restorative materials are identified, including the implementation of risk assessment in decision making.
- The specific clinical use of glass ionomer cement/resin-modified glass ionomer cement is presented.
- The specific clinical use of resin-based composite is presented.
- The specific clinical use of full-coverage stainless steel crowns is presented.

INTRODUCTION

Initiating preventive dentistry care for children, preferably beginning no later than the age of 1 year, helps prevent dental caries.[1] Although it is ideal to strive for children to be caries free, data indicate that 70% of children have experienced at least 1 cavitated carious lesion by age 17.[2] Many children, particularly children at high risk for dental caries, still experience cavitated lesions in both the primary and permanent dentitions.

Using the concept of minimally invasive dentistry, restoration placement is a last resort when prevention of a cavitated lesion has failed. Teeth can be restored using a minimally invasive restorative protocol with restorative materials that most appropriately meet the needs of the patient, risk assessment, age of the patient, size of the cavitated lesion, and ability to isolate the cavity preparation all being important considerations.

GLASS IONOMER CEMENT/RESIN-MODIFIED GLASS IONOMER CEMENT

Fluoride release occurs during the glass ionomer cement setting reaction and continues at low fluoride release levels for years.[3,4] There is an advantage of using glass ionomer cement restorations in children that are at moderate risk for the development of caries or secondary caries because the fluoride associated with the glass ionomer restorative materials can inhibit tooth demineralization at the restoration cavosurface margin.[5–7]

Department of Developmental Dentistry, Dental School, University of Texas Health Science Center at San Antonio, 7703 Floyd Curl Drive, San Antonio, TX 78229-3900, USA
E-mail address: donly@uthscsa.edu

Dent Clin N Am 57 (2013) 75–82
http://dx.doi.org/10.1016/j.cden.2012.09.001
0011-8532/13/$ – see front matter © 2013 Elsevier Inc. All rights reserved.

Occlusal Restorations

Occlusal glass ionomer cement restorations have shown clinical success.[8–10] Contemporary heavily filled glass ionomer cements and resin-modified glass ionomer cements have compressive strengths that provide adequate wear properties for the posterior primary dentition. Glass ionomer would be considered for occlusal restorations when there might be difficulty in isolating a tooth to keep it dry enough for the placement of a resin-based composite restoration.

Class II Restorations

Class II resin-modified glass ionomer cement restorations have shown clinical success.[8–12] The advantage of not needing to acid-etch tooth structure before restoration placement and knowing the glass ionomer chemical reaction will occur even with mild saliva contamination, makes the material favorable for the pediatric patient, in whom speed is critical and tooth isolation difficult.

Preparation design for class II glass ionomer cement restorations in the primary dentition is similar to amalgam preparations. The proximal box should be deep enough to break contact, and the axial wall should ideally extend 1.25 mm. The lateral walls should slightly converge to the occlusal, which aids in mechanical retention of the restorative material. The proximal box buccal and lingual walls should remain within the line angles of the tooth; breaking buccal or lingual contact is not necessary. No cavosurface bevels are placed in glass ionomer cement preparations because glass ionomer cement is brittle and could easily break or chip at beveled cavosurface beveled margins. After preparation, a matrix band or T-band is placed interproximally and wedged firmly so that the restorative material can be placed and adapted into the cavity preparation, and an adequate contact point can be created with the adjacent tooth.

Class III Restorations

Class III glass ionomer cement restorations have shown clinical success.[9,10] These glass ionomer cement restorations would be indicated when perfect isolation for a resin-based composite restoration is not possible. Lingual access for maxillary anterior teeth and labial access for mandibular anterior teeth is appropriate for class III preparations.

Class V Restorations

Class V glass ionomer cement restorations have shown clinical success in the primary dentition.[9,10] Glass ionomer cement/resin-modified glass ionomer cement class V restorations are indicated when good isolation of the tooth is difficult or impossible for the placement of a resin-based composite restoration.

The Class V glass ionomer preparation design extends 1.25 mm pulpally, unless caries progresses further. No bevels are placed on the cavosurface margin because of the brittle nature of glass ionomer cement and potential for fracture at a beveled cavosurface margin.

Interim Therapeutic Restoration

The *interior therapeutic restoration* is the current term used in place of the initially introduced term *atraumatic restorative technique*. Atraumatic restorative technique was introduced in areas in which contemporary air-driven hand pieces and suction were not readily available.[13] Hand instruments were used to remove caries, then chemically cured glass ionomer cement was placed as a restorative material. This technique originated for use in third-world countries, where access to dental care was difficult.[14]

Today, the interim therapeutic restoration is thought to be more descriptive of the procedures performed, particularly in the United States.

RESIN-BASED COMPOSITE
Occlusal Restorations

Resin-based composite is the restorative material of choice for occlusal restorations when the tooth can be adequately isolated.[15,16] The wear and compressive strength of currently available resin-based composites have shown clinical success for occlusal and class II posterior restorations.

Occlusual preparations extend as far as caries progresses. Cavosurface margins are beveled, and heavily filled resins are used to withstand occlusal stress and wear. Any pits and fissures not included in the preparation can have sealant placed to prevent the development of future caries. Enamel should be acid etched with 35%–40% phosphoric acid for 15–30 seconds[17] and thoroughly rinsed, then a resin adhesive placed according to the manufacturer's instructions.[18,19] If the preparation extends well into dentin, a glass ionomer cement base can be used to replace dentin, then a heavily filled resin-based composite should be placed in 2-mm increments to ensure that the material is polymerized adequately.[20] Restorations are finished and polished and a final adhesive is then placed to fill in any imperfections created during finishing and to reach maximum polymerization at the restoration surface.[21,22]

Class II Restorations

Class II resin-based composite has shown clinical success.[15,16,23–28] The American Dental Association Statement on Posterior Resin-Based Composites reports that recommendations for class II restorations were for preparations that did not include restoration margins exhibiting heavy occlusal wear,[29] that is, restorations that do not extend beyond the line angles of the tooth or approximately one-half the intercuspal distance.

The class II resin-based composite preparation design is similar to that of the class II glass ionomer cement preparation in the primary dentition (**Fig. 1**). The main difference is that a cavosurface bevel is placed on all enamel margins in a resin-based composite preparation.[16] The proximal box should ideally just break gingival contact; the buccal and lingual walls should be within the line angles and converge toward the occlusal. There should be an occlusal extension from the proximal box that dovetails into the occlusal surface to provide additional retention. A matrix or T-band is placed interproximally and firmly wedged to achieve an adequate restoration contact point. After bevel

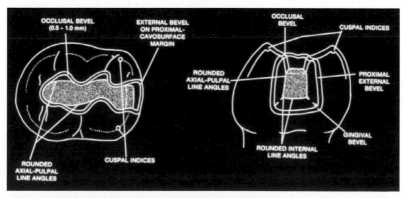

Fig. 1. The preparation design for a primary mandibular second molar class II resin-based composite restoration.

placement on cavosurface margins, the tooth is acid etched with 35%–40% phosphoric acid for 15–30 seconds; the chosen adhesive should be placed according to manufacturer's instructions, and resin-based composite is then placed and polymerized in 2-mm increments. The matrix is removed and the restoration is finished and polished, followed by the placement of an adhesive over the polished surface of the restoration.

Class III Restorations

Class III resin-based restorations have shown clinical success and have been recommended for the primary and permanent dentitions.[15,16] These restorations are appropriate for anterior teeth that can be adequately isolated to prevent contamination during restoration placement. The incisal edge should be intact after preparation to adequately retain the resin-based composite. Patients considered at high-risk for future caries development may be better served with more aggressive treatment, such as placement of full tooth coverage restorations.[30] Lingual preparation access is recommended for maxillary anterior teeth and labial preparation access is recommended for mandibular anterior teeth. The box of the preparation should extend to where caries has progressed, and all enamel cavosurface margins should be beveled. Resin-based composite is then placed in 2-mm increments and polymerized and the restorations finished and polished as previously described.

Class IV Restorations

Class IV resin-based composite restorations have been recommended for the primary and permanent dentions.[15,16] Although class IV restorations would be unusual in the primary dentition, because in most circumstances a strip crown would be appropriate, there may be circumstances in which minimal enamel is chipped and a resin can be placed. Class IV resin-based composite restorations in the permanent anterior dentition have been recommended as an esthetic and effective restoration.[15,16] Contemporary highly filled resin-based composites offer greater strength to restorations than the lower-filled resins used traditionally. Because of this increased strength, a beveled chamfer preparation can offer additional bond strength to prevent fracture at the margin of the restoration.[31]

Class V Restorations

Class V resin-based composite restorations have been recommended for the primary and permanent dentions.[15,16] Isolation is critical to prevent contamination of the acid-etched preparations during restoration placement. Cavity preparation should extend only as far as caries has progressed. Ideally, the axial wall would extend 1.25 mm, and all internal walls should be rounded. Mechanical retention is created naturally with the use of a #330 bur. Enamel cavosurface margins should be beveled. A glass ionomer liner/base can be placed over prepared dentin, or a dentin adhesive can be placed over prepared dentin following manufacturer's instructions. Enamel margins are acid etched with 35%–40% phosphoric acid for 15–30 seconds, adhesive is applied according to manufacturer's instructions, and then resin-based composite is placed and polymerized in 2-mm increments. Finishing and polishing is accomplished as previously discussed.

Strip Crown Restorations

Bonded resin-based composite strip crowns have been recommended for the restorations of multiple-surface carious primary incisors.[32,33] Adequate tooth structure is necessary after cavity preparation to support the bonding of a strip crown.[34] Gingival health is also important when placing strip crowns. Gingivitis leads to bleeding at pressure contact; therefore, the pressure created by the celluloid strip crown forms can cause bleeding.

Preparation design for strip crowns includes reduction of the incisal edge 1.5 mm, reduction of proximal surfaces 1.0–1.5 mm with tapering toward the incisal edge, then placement of a labial-incisal and lingual-incisal bevel.[35]

The appropriate celluloid crown is then selected. The natural mesiodistal width of the unprepared tooth is the easiest dimension to use when selecting the appropriate celluloid crown size. The gingival margin of the celluloid crown can be cut with scissors to adapt to the natural free gingival margin.[36] The prepared tooth structure is then acid-etched with 35%–40% phosphoric acid for 15–30 seconds. Bonding adhesive is applied according to manufacturer's instructions, and then a celluloid crown that has been approximately half filled with resin-based composite is fit onto the prepared tooth (**Fig. 2**). The recommendation is to place a small hole in the incisal edge of the celluloid crown form so that excess resin can extrude through the hole. This method relieves the creation of air voids within the strip crown resin. Excess resin is removed from the gingival margin and the incisal edge of the celluloid crown, and then the resin is polymerized from both the facial surface and lingual surface. The celluloid crown form is peeled away, and there should be minimal finishing and polishing needed. Occlusion should be checked to see that the restoration is in normal occlusion and does not have premature incisal contact.

STAINLESS STEEL CROWNS
Anterior

Esthetic stainless steel crowns
Several esthetic anterior primary stainless steel crowns (SSCs) are available in the marketplace. These esthetic SSCs are frequently referred to as *preveneered stainless steel crowns* (**Fig. 3**).[37,38] Indications for the placement of esthetic anterior SSCs include severe anterior caries, minimal tooth structure remaining secondary to

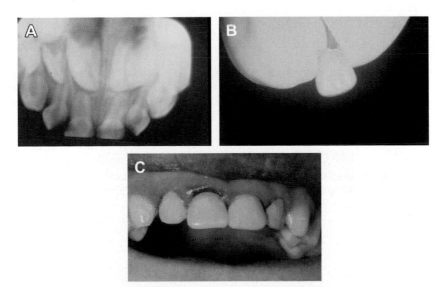

Fig. 2. (A) Radiograph of the maxillary primary incisors with severe caries indicating the need for full-coverage anterior restorations. (B) A trimmed celluloid crown form containing unpolymerized resin-based composite to fit to prepared incisors. (C) Final strip crown restorations.

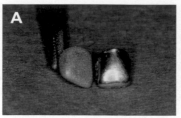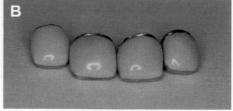

Fig. 3. (*A*) Maxillary anterior stainless steel crowns, one sandblasted in preparation for resin facing to be placed. (*B*) Maxillary anterior stainless steel crowns with following resin placement.

trauma, inability to isolate the tooth adequately for the placement of resin-based composite, and high risk for caries development.[33,39] Because of the uncooperative behavior of many children age 3 years or less, the esthetic SSCs may be the treatment of choice because placement is easier than the placement of resin-based composite (including strip crowns) and because perfect isolation of the tooth is not necessary.

There is potential for partial fracture or complete fracture of the resin veneered facial surface. Because of the physical properties associated with resin veneers over stainless steel, the resin has minimal flexure and can dislodge with the tensile and shear stress associated with typical mastication.[40]

SSC

Anterior SSCs have shown clinical success.[33,39] These crowns may not provide ideal esthetics, but they can be crimped on all gingival margins to obtain a well-adapted fit to tooth structure. In young children, in whom behavior frequently offers a challenging restorative process, and longevity of the restoration is critical, SSCs can be very effective restorations. The preparation design is similar to the preparation design for esthetic SSCs.

Posterior

SSC

Posterior SSCs have shown clinical success.[39,41] Indications for posterior SSC restorations include the inability to adequately isolate the tooth, expected longevity of multiple years, high caries risk, and posterior tooth restoration provided under general anesthesia.

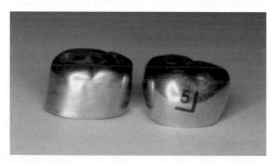

Fig. 4. Two types of commercially available posterior stainless steel crowns. The crown on the right is precrimped at the gingival margin.

Preparation design initiates with 1.5- to 2.0-mm occlusal reduction, followed by 1.0- to 1.5-mm converging proximal reduction. Line angles are then rounded, and a 45° level is placed at the occlusolabrial and occlusolingual margins. The prepared tooth now has an SSC fit. The gingival margin of the SSC is cut so that it extends subgingivally, but not to the extent of causing blanching at the periodontal ligament attachment. The adapted SSC margin is crimped and polished to snugly fit the tooth. Although some SSCs are precrimped, additional crimping may be necessary (**Fig. 4**). SSCs are cemented with glass ionomer cement or resin-modified glass ionomer cement, making sure the crown is completely seated and in normal occlusion.

REFERENCES

1. American Academy of Pediatric Dentistry. Definition of dental home. Pediatr Dent 2009;31(Special issue):10.
2. Vargas CM, Crall JJ, Scheider DA. Sociodemographic distribution of dental caries: NHANES III: 1988-1994. J Am Dent Assoc 1998;129:1229–38.
3. Forsten L. Fluoride release from a glass ionomer cement. Scand J Dent Res 1977; 85:503–4.
4. Olsen BT, Garcia-Godoy F, Marshall TD, et al. Fluoride release from glass ionomer-lined amalgam restorations. Am J Dent 1989;2:89–91.
5. Garcia-Godoy F, Jensen ME. Artificial recurrent caries in glass ionomer-lined amalgam restorations. Am J Dent 1990;3:89–93.
6. Griffin F, Donly KJ, Erickson R. Caries inhibition of fluoride-releasing liners. Am J Dent 1992;5:293–5.
7. Donly KJ, Segura A, Kanellis M, et al. Clinical performance and caries inhibition of resin-modified glass ionomer and amalgam restorations. J Am Dent Assoc 1999; 130:1459–66.
8. Croll TP, Bar-Zion Y, Segura A, et al. Clinical performance of resin-modified glass ionomer cement restorations in primary teeth. J Am Dent Assoc 2001;132: 1110–6.
9. Croll TP, Nicholson JW. Glass ionomer cements in pediatric dentistry: review of the literature. Pediatr Dent 2002;24:423–9.
10. Berg JH. Glass ionomer cements. Pediatr Dent 2002;24:430–8.
11. Vilkinis V, Horsted-Bindslev P, Baelum V. Two-year evaluation of class II resin-modified glass ionomer cement/composite open sandwich and composite restorations. Clin Oral Investig 2000;4:133–9.
12. Welbury RR, Shaw AJ, Murray JJ, et al. Clinical evaluation of paired compomer and glass ionomer restorations in primary molars: final results after 42 months. Br Dent J 2000;189:93–7.
13. Frencken JE, Songpaisan Y, Phantumvanit P, et al. An atraumatic restorative treatment (ART) technique: evaluation after 1 year. Int Dent J 1994;44:460–4.
14. Frencken JE, Makoni F, Sithole WD. Atraumatic restorative treatment and glass ionomer sealants in a school oral health programme in Zimbabwe: evaluation after 1 year. Caries Res 1996;30:428–33.
15. Burgess JO, Walker R, Davidson JM. Posterior resin-based composite: review of the literature. Pediatr Dent 2002;24:465–79.
16. Donly KJ, Garcia-Godoy F. The use of resin-based composite in children. Pediatr Dent 2002;24:480–8.
17. Redford DA, Clarkson BH, Jensen M. The effect of different etching times on the sealant bond strength, etch depth and pattern in primary teeth. Pediatr Dent 1986;8:11–5.

18. Swift EJ Jr. Dentin/enamel adhesives: review of the literature. Pediatr Dent 2002; 24:456–61.
19. Garcia-Godoy F, Donly KJ. Dentin/enamel adhesives in pediatric dentistry. Pediatr Dent 2002;24:462–4.
20. Caughman W, Rueggeberg F, Curtis J. Clinical guidelines for photocuring restorative resins. J Am Dent Assoc 1995;126:1280–6.
21. Simonsen RJ, Kanca J. Surface hardness of posterior composite resins using supplemental polymerization after simulated occlusual adjustment. Quintessence Int 1986;17:631–3.
22. Dickinson GL, Leinfelder KF. Assessing the long-term effect of a surface penetrating sealant. J Am Dent Assoc 1993;124:68–72.
23. Nelson GV, Osborne JW, Gale EN, et al. A three-year clinical evaluation of composite resin and a high copper amalgam in posterior primary teeth. ASDC J Dent Child 1980;47:414–8.
24. Oldenburg TR, Vann WF, Dilley DC. Composite restorations for primary molars: results after four years. Pediatr Dent 1987;9:136–43.
25. Tonn EM, Ryge G. Clinical evaluations of composite resin restorations in primary molars: a 4-year follow-up study. J Am Dent Assoc 1988;117:603–6.
26. Barnes DM, Blank LW, Thompson VP, et al. A 5-and 8-year clinical evaluation of a posterior composite resin. Quintessence Int 1991;22:143–51.
27. Barr-Agholme M, Oden A, Dahllof G, et al. A 2-year clinical study of light-cured composite and amalgam restorations in primary molars. Dent Mater 1991;7:230–3.
28. Attin T, Hartman O, Hildgers RD, et al. Fluoride retention of incipient enamel lesions after treatment with a calcium fluoride varnish in vivo. Arch Oral Biol 1995;40:169–74.
29. American Dental Association Council on Scientific Affairs and ADA Council on Dental Benefit Programs statement on posterior resin-based composites. J Am Dent Assoc 1998;129:1627–8.
30. Tinanoff N, Douglass JM. Clinical decision making for caries management in children. Pediatr Dent 2002;24:386–92.
31. Donly KJ, Browning R. Class IV preparation design for microfilled and macrofilled composite resin. Pediatr Dent 1992;14:34–6.
32. Lee JK. Restoration of primary anterior teeth: review of the literature. Pediatr Dent 2002;24:506–10.
33. Waggoner WF. Restoring primary anterior teeth. Pediatr Dent 2002;24:511–6.
34. Kupietzky A, Waggoner WF, Galea J. The clinical and radiographic success of bonded resin composite strip crowns for primary incisors. Pediatr Dent 2003; 25:577–81.
35. Webber DL, Epstein NB, Wong JW, et al. A method of restoring primary anterior teeth with the aid of a celluloid crown form and composite resins. Pediatr Dent 1979;1:244–6.
36. Grosso FC. Primary anterior strip crowns. J Pedod 1987;11:182–7.
37. Croll TP, Helpin M. Preformed resin-veneered stainless steel crowns for restoration of primary incisors. Quintessence Int 1996;27:309–13.
38. Croll TP. Primary incisor restorations using resin-veneered stainless steel crowns. ASDC J Dent Child 1998;65:89–95.
39. Seale NS. The use of stainless steel crowns. Pediatr Dent 2002;24:501–5.
40. Lin B. Aesthetic Crowns for the primary dentition. J Pediatr Dent Care 2005;11: 36–40.
41. Randall RC. Preformed metal crowns for primary and permanent molar teeth: review of the literature. Pediatr Dent 2002;24:489–500.

Pediatric Oral and Maxillofacial Surgery

Elizabeth Kutcipal, DDS

KEYWORDS

- Pediatric • Maxillofacial • Surgery • Craniofacial • Oral

KEY POINTS

- The procedures and techniques of oral and maxillofacial surgery (OMS) may be similar in adult and pediatric patients, but the behavioral and anesthetic considerations may be very different.
- Certain procedures and clinical findings may be more common in children, simply because of their age, growth, and development.
- Pediatric surgical patients should be evaluated as any other patient, with appropriate history, examination, and imaging.
- Surgical planning for pediatric patients should take into consideration age, behavior, dental and physiologic development, and maxillofacial growth.

INTRODUCTION

Pediatric patients are a special group of patients in the OMS practice. These patients can have a broad range of surgical needs, including, but not limited to, exodontia, soft-tissue surgery, treatment of pathology, fracture management, and orthognathic surgery. Many surgical procedures are similar on both adults and children. However, the frequency of the procedures may differ; for example, dental implants are rare in children and common in adults, just as mesiodens are common in children but rare in adults. Just as in adult patients, pediatric patients may have complex medical considerations; these patients may require treatment in a hospital setting. Although surgical technique may be similar in both pediatric and adult patients, pediatric patients should not be treated as "small adults." Pediatric patients have unique anesthetic, physiologic, and behavioral considerations. Surgical planning for pediatric patients must also take growth and development into consideration. Pediatric patients provide a unique challenge to the oral and maxillofacial surgeon, medically, physiologically, behaviorally, and perhaps surgically.

Seattle Children's Hospital, Department of Dentistry, 4800 Sandpoint Way, Seattle, WA 98109, USA
E-mail address: elizabeth.kutcipal@seattlechildrens.org

Dent Clin N Am 57 (2013) 83–98
http://dx.doi.org/10.1016/j.cden.2012.09.008
0011-8532/13/$ – see front matter © 2013 Elsevier Inc. All rights reserved.

DENTOALVEOLAR SURGERY

The most common pediatric OMS referral is for dentoalveolar surgery. Dental caries affects numerous pediatric patients. Unrestorable caries could result in the extraction of either primary or permanent teeth. Referrals for extraction of primary teeth are often a result of unmanageable behavior. The procedure may require an intravenous or general anesthetic. Despite advances in prevention and access to care, dental caries still affects many pediatric patients **Fig. 1**. Acutely infected teeth requiring extraction might also require incision and drainage with or without placement of a Penrose drain. Ankylosed primary teeth are problematic, in terms of space maintenance and management of proper dental eruption. Depending on the degree of ankylosis and submersion, these extractions can vary from simple to extremely difficult. Ankylosed primary teeth can often be managed by the pediatric dentist, but a referral may be warranted depending on the anticipated difficulty of the extraction (**Fig. 2**).

Another common pediatric patient referred to an OMS is for the extraction of supernumerary teeth. Supernumerary teeth can occur in any area but are common in the anterior maxilla. These teeth may present as a single entity or as several supernumerary teeth. Supernumerary teeth can cause failure of eruption of the permanent dentition or ectopic eruption of the permanent teeth. Several congenital syndromes present with multiple supernumerary teeth. An additional consideration would be orthodontic care that could not be accomplished because of the presence of the supernumerary teeth. Again, these extractions can range from simple to extremely difficult. Extensive soft-tissue flaps with bone removal may be required. More complex cases may warrant a cone beam computed tomographic (CT) scan for localization of the teeth (**Fig. 3**).

Third molars are also a common pediatric referral for an oral and maxillofacial surgeon. Early referrals may be due to pathology or the third molars preventing complete eruption of the second molars. More commonly, third molar referrals are a function of inadequate arch length, ectopic eruption, dental caries, pain, orthodontic movement, or pericoronitis. Referrals that indicate a reason may help the surgeon prioritize patient care. Patients preparing for orthognathic surgery may require removal of the mandibular third molars in anticipation of bilateral sagittal split osteotomy. Healing of this area before the mandibular osteotomy allows for a more predictable split of the mandible.[1]

Special considerations for dental extractions, including third molars, are those with complex medical or behavioral conditions. Patients undergoing chemotherapy may require removal if there is impending infection to avoid significant problems while severely immunocompromised. Hematology patients also require special consideration, depending on what blood products or pharmacologic management is

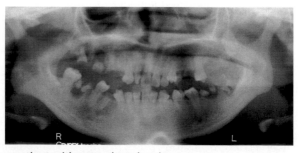

Fig. 1. A teenage patient with gross dental caries.

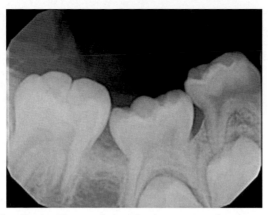

Fig. 2. A 7-year-old patient with an ankylosed primary second molar.

necessary. Many different bleeding disorders exist and should be managed in conjunction with the patient's hematologist. Patients who are nonverbal or completely uncooperative may undergo extractions while he/she is under general anesthesia for other issues, whether that is dental care, an ear, nose, and throat procedure, or so on.

Patients who are born with neonatal teeth may also require extraction at a young age. Neonatal teeth may be an aspiration risk or provide feeding challenges. Neonatal teeth also may be seen in patients with cleft lip and palate and require removal for pre-operative nasoalveolar molding. Some practioners accomplish these extractions with the use of topical anesthesia; it may be difficult to assess the amount of topical anesthesia administered given the infant's weight. Often, several drops of local anesthesia injected into the soft-tissue stalk of the neonatal tooth provide local anesthesia and hemostasis for the extraction. The calcified portion of the neonatal tooth should be removed in addition to the soft-tissue stalk. Hemostasis is an important consideration and can generally be managed with direct pressure.[2]

Ectopically erupting teeth also generate surgical referrals. These teeth may be indicated for extraction if they are extremely misguided. Orthodontists may request "exposure and bonding" of impacted teeth for forced orthodontic eruption. Maxillary canines are common referrals for exposure and bonding, but many other teeth in the arch can require forced orthodontic eruption as well. Teeth that have been blocked from eruption, such as by a supernumerary tooth or odontoma may need orthodontic traction to aid eruption. Orthodontic involvement is paramount and required when

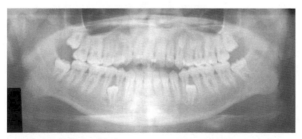

Fig. 3. A teenage patient with multiple supernumerary teeth.

dealing with forced eruption of teeth. Communication between the providers is essential for an ideal outcome (**Fig. 4**).[3]

Soft-tissue procedures are also referral requests. Lingual or labial frenectomies are common requests. A lingual frenectomy may be requested early in life for feeding issues or speech difficulties due to tongue immobility. Ankyloglossia is sometimes managed by the pediatrician if identified to be problematic in infancy. Frena with high attachment may have periodontal impacts on the adjacent teeth. The high muscle attachments of a maxillary frenum may create a diastema between the teeth. This is a normal finding in young patients. A frenectomy may be required to orthodontically close the diastema and avoid relapse in this area.

Dentoalveolar procedures are common in the pediatric population. Referrals to oral and maxillofacial surgeons are generally for more complex surgical dentoalveolar procedures or for patients with medical or behavioral complexities.

TRAUMA

Pediatric patients are not immune to maxillofacial trauma. Trauma may involve simple dental trauma, including dental fractures or luxation of both primary and permanent teeth. Most pediatric dentists are comfortable managing these isolated dental injuries. A more extensive injury would be a dentoalveolar fracture, which involves a fracture of the underlying bony alveolus, with or without luxation of the dentition. This condition is often managed by rigid splinting, or perhaps extraction of teeth, if necessary. Pediatric patients can sustain mandibular fractures for a variety of reasons, including sports injuries, motor vehicle crashes, and assault. These fractures have a variety of treatment modalities, depending on the age of the patient and the location of the fractures. Careful questioning about the mechanism of injury and concomitant injuries is imperative. Loss of consciousness should be assessed in all patients with suspected facial fractures. Loss of consciousness could be an indication of underlying intracranial injury and should be referred appropriately.

Mandibular fractures can occur in the mandibular symphysis (midline), mandibular parasymphysis (between the mandibular canines), mandibular body, mandibular angle, or mandibular condyle (either through the condylar neck or through the joint itself). Multiple mandibular fractures are not uncommon. Treatment of mandibular fractures ranges from nonsurgical treatment to open reduction and internal fixation of the injuries. Nonsurgical treatment generally involves a modified diet and close follow-up. Open reduction with internal fixation involves the use of surgical plates to stabilize a fracture. A custom, prefabricated splint may be useful in patients who have multiple mandibular fractures to stabilize one fracture but allow for movement

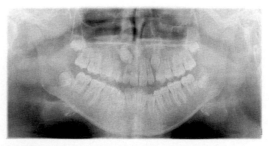

Fig. 4. A 13-year-old patient with impacted maxillary canines.

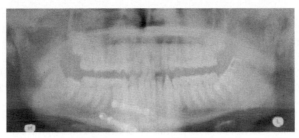

Fig. 5. A 16-year-old patient status post open reduction and internal fixation of bilateral mandibular fractures.

of the mandible if temporomandibular joint (TMJ) ankylosis is a concern. Young children are rarely placed in maxillomandibular fixation for intracapsular mandibular condylar factures because of the risk of TMJ ankylosis. When examining a patient with a suspected mandibular fracture, the patient should be assessed for malocclusion, bony instability, numbness of the lip/chin, gingival tearing, floor of mouth ecchymosis, and radiographic findings consistent with a fracture. Children who sustain mandibular factures require short-term follow-up for the acute injury and long-term follow-up to assess for growth disturbances as a result of the fracture (**Fig. 5**).[4]

Other bony fractures can occur in pediatric patients as well. Midfacial fractures, such as LeFort fractures (I, II, III) or zygomaticomaxillary fractures, can occur in pediatric patients but are less common because of the development of the facial sinuses. Nasal fractures can also occur in pediatric patients, although often these fractures do not require intervention. Direct blows to the orbital region can cause orbital blowout fractures, which are fractures of the orbital floor. Orbital injuries are of concern if there is injury to the globe itself or if the orbital contents become entrapped within the fracture edges. This generally means that the patient is unable to gaze upward, because the inferior rectus muscle is trapped within the fracture. If not recognized, this can lead to permanent limitation of eye movement. Entrapment can be recognized by

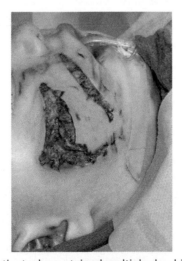

Fig. 6. An 18-month-old patient who sustained multiple dog bites.

limitations in upward gaze, nausea, or bradycardia due to the oculocardiac reflex. Suspected orbital injuries should be evaluated by an ophthalmologist, pediatrician, or emergency physician, at minimum.[5]

Children can also sustain soft-tissue injuries, which may be isolated or in combination with bony injury. Intraoral tissues may be lacerated because of falls, foreign objects, and so on. Often the gingival tissue is torn when an underlying mandibular fracture is present. The skin of the face is also a common area for laceration, again, from falls, direct trauma, or animal bites. Animal bites should be evaluated by a medical provider to discuss the need for a tetanus booster, rabies coverage, and antibiotic coverage (**Fig. 6**).[6]

Children suffer facial injuries with some frequency, largely as a result of their activities. Injuries can range from small dental injuries to panfacial fractures. Patients should be evaluated for concomitant injuries. Dental injuries can often be managed in a dental office, but more significant injuries should be referred appropriately.

PATHOLOGY

Pediatric patients present with a variety of pathologic conditions in the oral cavity. Lesions can range from soft-tissue to bony lesions and benign cysts to malignant tumors. Most of the pathologic conditions identified in pediatric patients are benign, but diagnosis should be confirmed by analysis of a pathologic specimen. Most surgeons would agree that anomalous tissue that is removed should be sent for pathologist review. Practitioners may be tempted to give a diagnosis based on differential diagnosis; however, gross review of a lesion does not substitute for a microscopic review. Parents of patients are anxious for a diagnosis and often need to be reminded that the pathology needs to be reviewed to find the answer.

A common soft-tissue lesion in pediatric patients is a mucocele, or mucous extravasation phenomenon. Often, these resolve spontaneously. Lesions that are frequently traumatized, however, are unlikely to resolve spontaneously. Generally, these are thought to be due to injury to the duct of the minor salivary gland, causing a fluid collection in that area. These injuries can be difficult to manage. Removal and biopsy of the mucocele provides a definitive diagnosis. Large lesions can be a social stigma, especially as patients this age enter school. Recurrence is a definite possibility, due to iatrogenic injury of the surrounding minor salivary glands/ducts, habitual injury by the patient, injury by orthodontic appliances, or accidental injury of the area while it is still affected by local anesthesia. A location-specific mucocele is a ranula, which is found in the floor of the mouth. The cause for this entity is injury to the sublingual duct, causing an accumulation of fluid in this area. These injuries often look bluish, as a result of the fluid accumulation. Ranulas can be superficial in the floor of the mouth or plunging, implying that they are below the mylohyoid muscle. Plunging ranulas can grow and expand into the tissues of the neck; these are treated by marsupialization of the ranula or by complete removal of the sublingual gland. Some practitioners advocate marsupialization, as it is less invasive and has less risk to the anatomy in the area. The disadvantage of marsupialization is that the ranula may recur (**Fig. 7**).[3]

Another common soft-tissue lesion in children is the pyogenic granuloma. This lesion can present in a variety of ways, from small and benign-looking to large and ulcerated. Pyogenic granuloma can be due to trauma or a foreign body in the area, such as cement from an orthodontic appliance or space maintainer. These lesions are vascular and have a propensity to bleed when manipulated or surgically removed. Larger lesions may be ulcerated with areas of necrosis and a fetid odor. Larger lesions may look similar to malignant lesions (**Fig. 8**).[7]

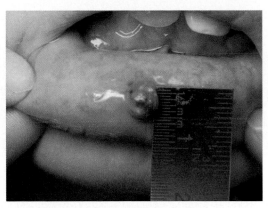

Fig. 7. An 8-year-old girl with a mucocele of the lower lip.

Odontomas are lesions of the enamel and dentin, often seen in children. These lesions are made of enamel and dentin but are not formed in the shape of a normal tooth. Odontomas may be compound or complex. The compound odontoma looks like multiple miniature teeth. The complex odontoma generally looks like a large mass of enamel and dentin. These lesions are problematic, because they often prevent the eruption of normal teeth. The odontoma may also represent the malformation of the tooth that should be in that area. If this is the case, the patient will then be missing that tooth. These lesions can grow to be large but are generally asymptomatic (**Fig. 9**).[7]

Dentigerous cysts are common in pediatric patients. These cysts can be benign appearing as a large-looking dental follicle. They may also manifest as a large lesion associated with an impacted tooth. Although benign, these lesions can grow to be large. They may move teeth but rarely resorb teeth. They are treated by surgical removal. These lesions are not infrequent in pediatric patients (**Fig. 10**).

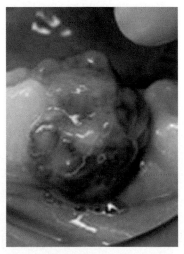

Fig. 8. An 11-year-old girl with a large pyogenic granuloma in the left mandible.

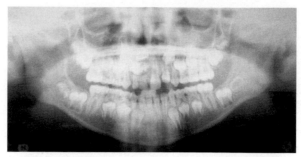

Fig. 9. An 8-year-old girl with a large odontoma of the anterior maxilla.

A buccal infected cyst is a bony lesion in children that is generally seen around erupting mandibular permanent first molars. Patients can present with bony expansion adjacent to an erupting mandibular first permanent molar. Frank purulence may or may not be present. Radiographically, there is a saucer-like appearance around the affected tooth. This condition is treated with surgical curettage of the area and generally resolve once the tooth has completely erupted.[8]

Idiopathic bone cavity is an entity often seen in pediatric patients. Previously, idiopathic bone cavities were called "traumatic bone cavities" or "hemorrhagic bone cysts." These names are misleading because the cause is unknown, and the lesions have no epithelial lining. This lesion presents as a radiolucency in the mandible, is not associated with an impacted tooth, and can be small or large. Biopsy and exploration is indicated to make a definitive diagnosis. Radiographs and CT scans cannot effectively diagnose this lesion. Intraoperatively, opening this bony cavity reveals an empty hole, with no epithelial lining. Adequate exposure is necessary to ensure that no epithelium is inadvertently missed. A bony cavity, with no epithelial lining is pathognomonic for an idiopathic bone cavity (**Fig. 11**).

Ameloblastomas are rare in the pediatric population but not unheard of. The mean age for the occurrence of solid ameloblastomas is in the third to seventh decade of life. Unicystic ameloblastomas have a slightly lower mean age (second decade) but are still a rare entity in the pediatric population (**Fig. 12**).[7] Similarly, calcifying odontogenic epithelial tumors (Pindborg tumors) are found in a similar age group but can occasionally be seen in the pediatric population (**Fig. 13**).[9]

Central giant cell lesions are common in pediatric patients. They present as a radiolucent lesion in the mandible. They are often multilocular without an associated

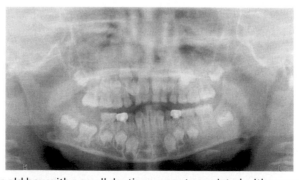

Fig. 10. A 7-year-old boy with a small dentigerous cyst associated with unerupted tooth #30.

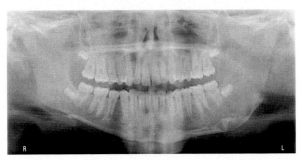

Fig. 11. A large idiopathic bone cavity of the left mandible in a 12-year-old girl.

impacted tooth. These lesions are unique, in that they may cross the mandibular midline. Giant cell lesions can also range in size from small and minimally aggressive to large and aggressive. Treatment of these lesions is variable, from enucleation to resection and with or without the use of adjunctive treatments, depending on many factors (eg, size, aggressiveness, and location).[10]

Melanotic neuroectodermal tumors of infancy are a rare lesion but limited to the pediatric population. These tumors often occur in the anterior maxilla but may be found in the mandible or other remote locations. The infant often has an asymptomatic swelling and expansion, which may be apparent by gross visualization or by difficulty feeding because of the size of the lesion. Surgical removal is required. Close follow-up is mandatory, as these lesions have a 15% recurrence rate (**Fig. 14**).[11]

Odontogenic keratocysts (OKCs) or keratocystic odontogenic tumors are not infrequent in children. The mean age for the occurrence of these lesions is in the 20s; however, they may be seen in younger patients. They occur in either the mandible or the maxilla and are often associated with an impacted tooth. These lesions are characterized by a thin lining, which, histologically, is only 6 to 8 cells thick. Treatment of these lesions varies depending on the surgeon. Some recommend careful and complete removal of the cystic lining. Others recommend this treatment, plus treatment of the bony cavity with either liquid nitrogen or Carnoy's solution. Still others advocate surgical resection. Patients who have basal cell nevus syndrome (Gorlin syndrome) tend to have multiple OKCs. They should be monitored frequently for new, or possibly recurrent, lesions. These lesions, regardless of syndromic association, can recur. After removal of these lesions, patients should be on long-term follow-up to evaluate for new lesions (**Fig. 15**).[12]

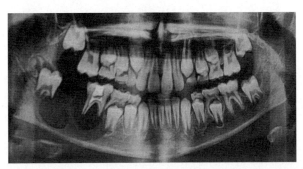

Fig. 12. A 9-year-old boy with a unicystic ameloblastoma of the right mandible.

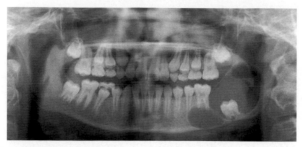

Fig. 13. A CEOT of the left mandible in an 11-year-old girl.

Ameloblastic fibroma is a lesion seen in the pediatric population, most often in the first or second decade of life. It generally occurs in the posterior mandible and is often associated with an unerupted tooth. As with many of the lesions mentioned, long-term follow-up is essential. These lesions can recur, with possible recurrence as an ameloblastic fibrosarcoma (**Fig. 16**).[13]

Fibrous dysplasia is a lesion that may affect one bone or several bones: monostotic versus polyostotic. Fibrous dysplasia can have a syndromic association with McCune-Albright syndrome. Although it is a benign entity, the change in the bony architecture can be dramatic. Patients may develop significant asymmetry associated with fibrous dysplasia. Confirming the diagnosis is important for ongoing care. Radiographically, bone has a ground glass appearance. Histologically, fibrous dysplasia has the appearance of Chinese characters. These lesions are generally followed clinically and rarely grow after puberty the patient has reached their twenties. Fibrous dysplasia may require surgical treatment if it is significantly deforming or affects adjacent anatomic structures (**Figs. 17** and **18**).[10]

Osteosarcoma of the facial bones is a rare lesion in pediatric patients. Osteoscarcoma of the long bones is much more common. Generally, patients with osteosarcoma of the facial bones are in the third decade of life. A pediatric patient with an osteosarcoma of the facial bones should be treated in combination with the

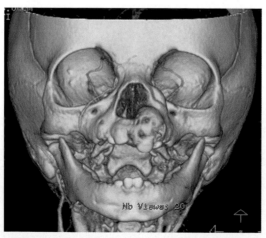

Fig. 14. A 3-dimensional CT scan of a melanotic neuroectodermal tumor of infancy in a 6-month-old boy.

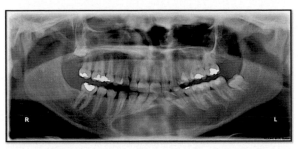

Fig. 15. A large odontogenic keratocyst (KOT) in a teenager with basal cell nevus syndrome.

medical center's tumor board and oncology service. A full workup would provide information for determining treatment of this patient, whether surgery or chemotherapy plus surgery, in addition to the reconstructive options (**Fig. 19**).[14]

Pediatric patients can have a large variety of cysts and tumors of the craniofacial region. A sampling of benign lesions was discussed in this article, but there are many more. Although rare, malignant lesions may present in the oral cavity, such as Ewing's sarcoma, leukemia, rhabdomyosarcoma, and Burkitt's lymphoma. Treatment can vary from aggressive resection to nonoperative intervention. Definitive diagnosis via histopathologic review is imperative. A common theme throughout this section is the need for long-term follow-up and appropriate referral, which is true for most pathologic conditions.

CONGENITAL ANOMALIES
Cleft Lip and Palate

Providers dealing with pediatric patients are bound to see patients with congenital anomalies. One of the most common anomalies seen is cleft lip and palate. Different populations and ethnic groups have different incidences of cleft lip and palate. These anomalies can present as isolated cleft lip, isolated cleft palate, or unilateral/bilateral cleft lip and palate. Clefts can range from incomplete clefts to large, deforming clefts. Each patient has individual, unique treatment needs. Patients with an isolated cleft palate are more likely to have an associated syndrome. A general timeline of treatment is planned for these patients; these interventions may vary depending on the geographic location, the surgeon, and the concomitant medical issues of the patient.

The primary lip repair is generally performed at 3 to 4 months of age. Some infants with cleft lip may undergo nasoalveolar molding or lip taping before the surgical repair.

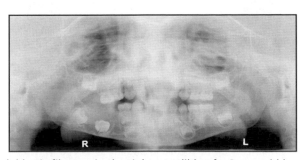

Fig. 16. An ameloblastic fibroma in the right mandible of a 3-year-old boy.

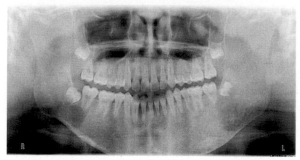

Fig. 17. Fibrous dysplasia in the left mandible of a teenage boy. Notice the ground glass appearance.

The "rule of tens" is generally considered when infants require general anesthesia: 10 pounds, 10 weeks of age, and a hemoglobin of 10 g/dL. This rule helps to dictate the safety of the anesthesia for the infant. The primary palate repair is generally done in about 8 to 14 months of age, but this can greatly vary from center to center. Palate repair is based on the development of speech. An intact palate is ideal for the child to begin to develop their first words. There are several different palate repair techniques, the details of which are not discussed here.

Patients with clefts often have speech issues related to the length of the soft palate and orientation of the musculature of the soft palate. At age 4 or 5 years, a speech pathologist can perform a diagnostic speech examination. Should the patient have anatomic issues with speech difficulties, often velopharyngeal insufficiency, a secondary speech procedure, such as a Furlow palatoplasty, pharyngoplasty, or pharyngeal flap, may be necessary.

Patients with clefting that includes the maxillary alveolus require bone grafting to make the maxilla a unified entity. This bone grafting occurs usually between the ages of 6 and 12 years. Timing for the alveolar bone graft is generally based on the

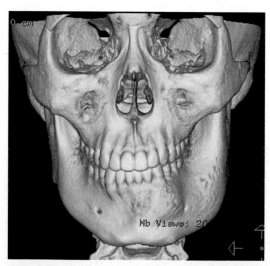

Fig. 18. A 3-dimensional CT scan of the same patient as in **Fig. 17** with fibrous dysplasia; notice the expansion of his mandible.

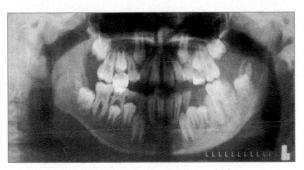

Fig. 19. Osteosarcoma of the left mandible in a 10-year-old boy.

development of the permanent maxillary canine or the presence of a lateral incisor. An oronasal communication may also be present. If a lateral incisor is present, the bone graft is completed earlier to maintain bony support for the lateral incisor as it erupts. If the lateral incisor is absent, the bone graft is completed when the maxillary canine root development is approximately half complete. Autogenous grafting is generally obtained from the anterior iliac crest. There are several other sites from where bone can be obtained, but the iliac crest is one of the most used. Bone morphogenic protein has been used by some for alveolar bone grafting. This procedure aims to create a complete alveolus and to close remaining oronasal/palatal communications (**Fig. 20**).

Patients with cleft lip and palate often develop maxillary hypoplasia as they grow, likely due to the extensive surgical procedures they have undergone before growth cessation, involving stripping of periosteum. Orthodontics in combination with orthognathic surgery occurs for correction of the underlying malocclusion. The patient may require LeFort I osteotomy for the advancement of the maxilla and may or may not require mandibular setback. Depending on the amount of maxillary advancement, a bone graft may be considered to help aid in long-term stability.[15]

Pierre Robin Sequence

Patients with Pierre Robin sequence may or may not require surgical intervention. These patients have the triad of micrognathia, cleft palate, and glossoptosis. This condition may be part of Stickler syndrome, which also carries the diagnosis of high myopia. The mandible is often extremely small and may have respiratory impacts on the infant. These infants often require careful positioning to maintain a patent airway. If positioning is not effective, a nasopharyngeal airway may be warranted. More aggressive interventions may be required, such as mandibular distraction to

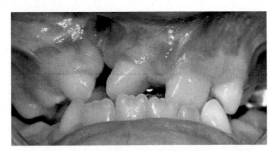

Fig. 20. Intraoral view of a patient with cleft in the mixed dentition.

increase the airway space or tracheostomy. The cleft of the palate is often described as "U-shaped." The thought is that the small size of the mandible forces the tongue into the palate region in utero, so the palatal shelves are unable to completely close. These clefts may be narrow or wide. Repair of these clefts can be challenging because of the size of the cleft and the potential for concomitant airway obstruction.

Other Craniofacial Conditions

Oral and maxillofacial surgeons come across a myriad of other craniofacial conditions, including, but are not limited to, Crouzon syndrome, Apert syndrome, amniotic band syndrome, Kabuki syndrome, and Pfeiffer syndrome. These patients may need routine dentoalveolar surgery. They also may require corrective orthognathic surgery to idealize their occlusion. Each patient clearly has unique needs that should be evaluated on a case-by-case basis.

ORTHOGNATHIC SURGERY

A common referral to oral and maxillofacial surgeons is for orthognathic surgery. This referral is generally generated from an orthodontist, because treatment is a combination of orthodontics and surgery. Orthodontic decompensation in preparation for orthognathic surgery takes about 12 to 18 months, if all goes as planned. Orthognathic surgery is completed with the orthodontic appliances in place. A surgical wire, surgical hooks, and molar bands are placed in preparation for surgery. A brief hiatus is taken from active orthodontic treatment to allow for healing after surgery. Most surgeons recommend a modified diet and limited activity for approximately 6 weeks after surgery. Orthodontic finishing is completed after surgery and takes 6 to 12 months for an ideal result.[16]

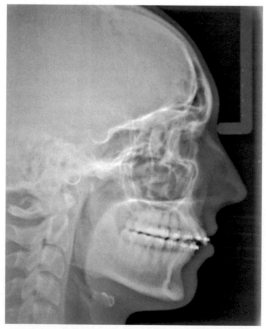

Fig. 21. Preoperative lateral cephalogram of a teenage patient with mandibular hypoplasia.

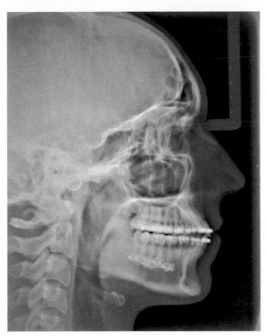

Fig. 22. Postoperative lateral cephalogram of the same patient as in Fig. 21 after bilateral sagittal split osteotomy.

Surgical correction may be required for multiple reasons. A patient may have a class II skeletal malocclusion, which can be corrected with a mandibular osteotomy for advancement. Routine mandibular advancements are generally done via bilateral sagittal split osteotomy; however, there are other mandibular osteotomies that may be used. A patient with a class III skeletal malocclusion may require a LeFort I osteotomy for advancement, mandibular osteotomy for setback, or a combination of the 2 procedures. Routine mandibular setback procedures are done using a bilateral sagittal split osteotomy; however, other surgical techniques may also be used. Most orthognathic surgery is completed using intraoral incisions, but some complicated cases require extraoral approaches (**Figs. 21** and **22**).

SUMMARY

Pediatric patients offer many challenges to oral and maxillofacial surgeons. The procedures and surgical technique may be similar in adult and pediatric patients, but the behavioral and anesthetic considerations are different. These patients have a subset of pathologic lesions that are unique to pediatric patients, and there are always exceptions to established norms. Certain procedures and clinical findings may be more common in children, simply because of their age, growth, and development. Pediatric surgical patients should be evaluated as any other patient, with appropriate history, examination, and imaging. Surgical planning for pediatric patients should take into consideration age, behavior, dental and physiologic development, and maxillofacial growth.

REFERENCES

1. Miloro M, Ghali G, Larsen P, et al. Peterson's principles of oral and maxillofacial surgery. Chapter 8: Impacted Teeth. 2004.

2. Cunha RF, Boer FA, Torriani DD, et al. Natal and neonatal teeth: review of the literature. Pediatr Dent 2001;23(2):158–62.
3. Kaban L, Troulis M. Pediatric oral and maxillofacial surgery. 2004:125–33, 152–58.
4. Goth S, Sawatari Y, Peleg M. Management of pediatric mandible fractures. J Craniofac Surg 2012;23(1):47–56.
5. Miloro M, Ghali G, Larsen P, et al. Peterson's principles of oral and maxillofacial surgery. 2004;24.
6. Presutti R. Prevention and treatment of dog bites. Am Fam Physician 2001;63(8): 1567–73.
7. Neville, Damm, Allen, et al. Oral and maxillofacial pathology. 1995;371–3, 513–9, 531–3.
8. Lim AA, Peck RG. Bilateral mandibular cyst: lateral radicular cyst, paradental cyst, or mandibular infected buccal cyst? Report of a case. J Oral Maxillofac Surg 2002;60:825–7.
9. Kaushal S, Mathur S, Vijay M, et al. Calcifying epithelial odontogenic tumor (Pindborg tumor) without calcification: a rare entity. J Oral Maxillofac Pathol 2012; 16(1):110–2.
10. Kaban L, Troulis M. Pediatric oral and maxillofacial surgery. 2004;216–23.
11. Johnson RE, Scheithauer BW, Dahlin DC. Melanotic neuroectodermal tumor of infancy a review of seven cases. Cancer 1983;52:661–6.
12. Li T. The odontogenic keratocyst: a cyst, or a cystic neoplasm. J Dent Res 2011; 90(2):1331–42.
13. Nelson B, Folk B. Ameloblastic fibroma. Head Neck Pathol 2009;3(1):51–3.
14. Neville, Damm, Allen, et al. Oral and maxillofacial pathology. 1995;482–85.
15. Posnick J. Craniofacial and maxillofacial surgery in children and young adults. 2000;32 and 33.
16. Profitt W, White R. Surgical-orthodontic treatment. 1991;7:226–47.

Temporomandibular Joint Disorders in Children

James A. Howard, DDS[a,b,*]

KEYWORDS

- Bruxism • Temporomandibular joint disorders • Internal derangement
- Facial asymmetry • Subluxation • Craniomandibular • Children • Adolescents

KEY POINTS

- Children seldom seek treatment for temporomandibular joint disorders (TMDs), but the dentist's awareness of the early signs and symptoms of TMD can facilitate quicker resolution and prevent progression. A child's difficulty in verbalizing the precise location and nature of facial pain and jaw dysfunction often results in a nondefinitive history, thus increasing the importance of the clinical evaluation.
- A focused examination of the masticatory musculature, the temporomandibular joints (TMJs), and associated capsular and ligamentous structures will reveal if a patient's headaches, otologic symptoms, or facial pains are TMD in origin.
- An accurate differential diagnosis enables timely referral to appropriate health care providers, reduces unnecessary consultations, and minimizes the use of diagnostic imaging. Completing a TMD screening history and examination can provide the clinician with the information needed to understand the possible causes and explain the child's condition.
- Guidelines on when to monitor TMDs or recommend treatment are not clearly established for children.

Children seldom seek treatment for temporomandibular joint disorders (TMDs), but the dentist's awareness of the early signs and symptoms of TMD can facilitate quicker resolution and prevent progression. A child's difficulty in verbalizing the precise location and nature of facial pain and jaw dysfunction often results in a nondefinitive history, thus increasing the importance of the clinical evaluation. A focused examination of the masticatory musculature, the temporomandibular joints (TMJs), and associated capsular and ligamentous structures will reveal if a patient's headaches,

Funding support: Center for Pediatric Dentistry, School of Dentistry, University of Washington.
Financial interests: The author has nothing to disclose.
[a] Center for Pediatric Dentistry, School of Dentistry, University of Washington, 6222 NE 74th St, Seattle, WA 98115, USA; [b] Temporomandibular Joint Dysfunction Clinic, Seattle Children's Hospital, 4800 Sand Point Way NE, Seattle, WA 98105, USA
* 720 North Evergreen Road, Suite 102, Spokane, WA 99216.
E-mail address: jhowarddds@hotmail.com

otologic symptoms, or facial pains are TMD in origin (**Box 1**). An accurate differential diagnosis enables timely referral to appropriate health care providers, reduces unnecessary consultations, and minimizes the use of diagnostic imaging. Completing a TMD screening history and examination can provide the clinician with the information needed to understand the possible causes and explain the child's condition. Guidelines for when to monitor TMDs or recommend treatment are not clearly established for children.

EPIDEMIOLOGY

A study of 3428 consecutive patients of all ages enrolled in a health maintenance organization who sought treatment for TMDs (**Fig. 1**) revealed that 85.4% were female.[1] The skewed age and gender distribution, compared with the general population of the United States (**Fig. 2**),[2] suggest a hormonal influence. Treatment-seeking peaks occur during the reproductive years, with a mean age of 33.8 years, and this must be taken into account when considering the validity of the proposed causes for TMDs.

The prevalence of signs and symptoms of TMD in children in population-based reports varies considerably.[3–5] The variation can be explained by the differences in the population investigated, by the examination methods and diagnostic criteria used, and by the interindividual and intraindividual variations of examiners.[6]

Gender differences in the prevalence of TMD are less evident in early childhood and become more accentuated between 15 and 50 years of age, but the female preponderance occurs at all ages. TMD pain in children increases with age in both girls

---

Box 1
TMDs: understanding and caring for your jaw problem

What are the signs and symptoms of a TMD?

Tenderness in the area in front of your ear, especially when you chew, speak, or open your mouth wide to sing or yawn.

Headache and discomfort in the muscles on the side of your face or head.

Clicking, popping, or grinding sounds when you open or close your mouth.

Difficulty opening your mouth wide and catching, sticking, or locking of the jaw.

Things you should do if you have a jaw problem

Apply moist heat and massage the muscles on the side of your face.

Take small bites or cut up food and place it between your back teeth. Avoid large foods that force you to open your mouth wide such as hamburgers and big sandwiches.

Avoid biting off food with your front teeth.

Eat soft foods such as yogurt, eggs, cereal, oatmeal, soup, and noodles.

Avoid chewy foods including licorice, beef jerky, bagels, taffy, gummy bears, bubble gum, French bread, and tough meats.

Avoid hard, crunchy foods such as raw vegetables, chips, and nuts.

Things you should not do when you have a jaw problem

Rest your hand on your chin when sitting at a desk or lying on the floor.

Play any wind instrument or violin or sing in a choir if these activities make your jaw hurt more.

Bite your fingernails or cuticles as this will aggravate your jaw joint and muscles.

Clench or grind your teeth. Remember to keep your lips together and your teeth apart.

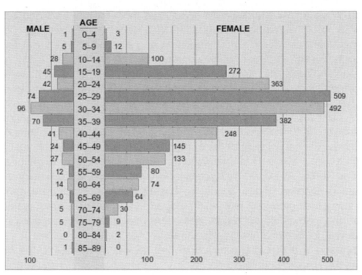

Fig. 1. Age and sex distribution of 3428 consecutive patients with TMD. (*Adapted from* Howard JA. Temporomandibular joint disorders, facial pain, and dental problems in performing artists. In: Satalott RT, Brandtonbrener AG, Lederman RJ, editors. Performing Arts Medicine. 3rd edition. Narberth (PA): Science & Medicine; 2010. p. 151–96.)

and boys.[7] Females with TMD pain seek care more often than males at all ages but the probability for someone seeking care for TMD correlates more strongly with an increase in the frequency and intensity of facial pain, regardless of age or sex.[8]

Wahlund and colleagues[9] reported that the prevalence of TMD in children and adolescents (12–18 years old) was 7%. Nilsson[10] found that the prevalence of TMD pain in 28,899 youths aged 12–19 years was 4.2% and was significantly higher in girls

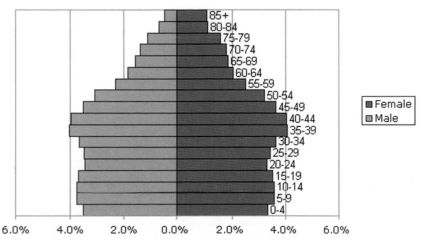

Fig. 2. Age and sex distribution of the US population in 2000. (*Data from* US Census Bureau. Statistical abstract of the United States: 2012. 131st edition. Washington, DC: US Census Bureau 2011.)

(6.0%) than boys (2.7%). Studies have correlated more frequent headaches and oto-logic symptoms[11,12] with the occurrence of TMD. Köhler and colleagues[13] concluded that the prevalence of severe TMD symptoms and signs in children and adolescents was generally low and did not change significantly during a 20-year follow-up period.

The Research Diagnostic Criteria for TMD (RDC/TMD),[14] used in many studies to define, standardize, and replicate the characteristics of the study samples, are useful in research analysis of groups of patients. The use of standardized diagnostic criteria for defining clinical subtypes of TMD as well as awareness that psychosocial factors are an important factor should lead to better treatment outcomes.[15] Dentists need to focus on the functional aspects of the dental occlusion, the biomechanical, or patho-physiologic aspects of the TMJ articulations, as well as the psychosocial aspects to best manage TMDs. As stated by Klasser and Green,[16] the word biopsychosocial is an excellent descriptor for the condition that TMD pain patients are living with, in that they have a biological problem which may activate pain pathways, with or without a demonstrable pathologic condition, and there may have been psychological ante-cedents as well as behavioral consequences.

A combination of physical and psychosocial factors contribute to the decision to seek treatment. For children, their parents' own experience with similar problems influ-ences this decision.[17,18] Of the 4262 consecutive patients with TMD seeking treatment in the private practice of the author during the past 15 years, 644 patients were less than 20 years of age (**Fig. 3**, **Table 1**), which represents 15.1% of all patients with TMD evaluated; whereas those less than 20 years of age represent 28.6% the general US population in 2000.[19]

Patients 15–19 years old account for 65.8 of the 644 patients (**Fig. 4**). No patients younger than 6 years of age were evaluated in last 15 years of private practice. Girls account for 89.9% of those over 15–19 years of age seeking treatment, and 75.5% of patients 6–14 years of age were female.

There are more male births than female births and until the age of 35 years, males represent a larger percentage of the US population.[20] The higher percentage of patients with TMD between the ages of 15 and 19 years and the increased ratio of females both suggest that different factors account for treatment-seeking behavior for TMD in young children than in adolescents. The impact of TMD pain on adolescents

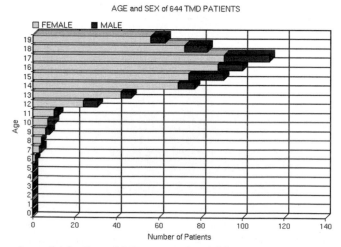

Fig. 3. Age and sex distribution of 644 consecutive children presenting with TMD.

Table 1
Age and sex distribution of 644 patients with TMD less than 20 years of age

	Age in Years																			
AGE	1	2	3	4	5	6	7	8	9	10	11	12	13	14	15	16	17	18	19
Male	0	0	0	0	0	0	1	0	2	3	2	7	5	8	17	12	22	11	7
Female	0	0	0	0	0	1	3	4	6	7	10	24	42	69	74	88	91	72	56
Total	0	0	0	0		1	4	4	8	10	12	31	47	77	91	100	113	83	63
% Male	/	/	/	/	/	/	25	0	25	30	17	23	11	10	18	12	19	13	11
% Female	/	/	/	/	/	/	100	75	100	75	70	83	77	89	90	82	88	81	87	89
Age as % of Total	/	/	/	/	/	/		.60	.60	1.2	1.5	1.9	4.8	7.4	12.0	14.1	15.5	17.7	12.9	9.8

differs by age and gender. A questionnaire was mailed to 350 clinic patients aged 12 to 19 years and 350 age-matched and sex-matched controls.[21] There were no age or sex differences in pain intensity, however for those adolescents aged 16–19 years, TMD pain had significantly greater impact on behavioral and psychosocial factors on girls than on boys. Among those aged 16 to 19 years, 32.4% of girls compared with 9.7% of boys reported school absences and analgesic consumption because of their TMD pain. This report is consistent with the finding of a significant increase in treatment seeking by girls aged 13 to 19 years (see **Table 1**).

Late adolescent patients with TMD had higher pain intensity in the orofacial region and reported more impact on activities of daily living, including difficulty in prolonged jaw opening, eating soft/hard foods, and sleeping, than younger patients. Of 167 patients age 16 to 18 years, girls reported significantly more problems than the boys due to headache and neck pain.[22]

ETIOLOGY

Greene[23] pointed out that the inability to identify precise causes or the lack of a perfect theoretical model does not prevent rendering sensible and often successful treatment of most patients with TMD. Historically, malocclusion has been considered a primary cause of TMD, but the occurrence of malocclusion, occlusal interferences, and

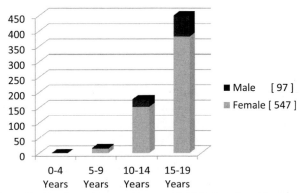

Fig. 4. Age and sex distribution of 644 patients with TMD less than 20 years of age by 5-year increments.

missing teeth is nearly equal for males and females.[24] However, most published studies evaluate static, morphologic variables and overlook the importance of the dynamic relationship between the joints and teeth during function. Restriction in the anterior envelope of function and dysfunctional occlusal contacts that alter the final path of closure during mastication both take on greater importance with the eruption of the permanent teeth. The increase in treatment seeking for TMD at 13 years of age (**Table 1**) coincides with full eruption of the second molars and the acceleration of growth of the mandible. Hormonal fluctuations in females have been implicated in altered pain perception and increased treatment seeking.[25–27] Micro and macro trauma[28] are known causes of TMD as are systemic factors[29] and disease.[30]

It is useful to categorize (**Table 2**) the causes as predisposing, precipitating and perpetuating.

Predisposing (or risk) factors for TMDs can be
- Systemic (affecting the entire body or a particular body system)
- Psychosocial (interaction of psychological and social variables)
- Physiologic (cellular and metabolic processes, neuromuscular)
- Structural (dental occlusion, musculoskeletal, articular, developmental anomalies).

Precipitating (or initiating) factors often involve trauma or overuse. Repetitive activities with the jaw in a sustained or abnormal posture or under abnormal load, such as when playing a wind instrument[31] or violin,[32,33] or sleep posture[34] can trigger a painful TMD episode.

Perpetuating (or sustaining) factors often include parafunction, overuse, systemic disease, occlusal factors, or psychological distress.[35,36]

Parafunction

Parafunctional activities are nonfunctional oromandibular activities that include jaw clenching, tooth grinding, tooth tapping, cheek biting, lip biting, and object biting occurring alone or in combinations. Bruxism is a movement disorder characterized by grinding and clenching of teeth (**Box 2**). Awake bruxism is found more in females than in males, whereas sleep bruxism (SB) shows no such sex prevalence. Data gathered from awake subjects cannot predict SB behavior and self-reports of bruxism during sleep are not reliable. Cause of bruxism has been reported in 3 categories: psychosocial factors, peripheral occlusal factors, and neurophysiologic factors. Most SB episodes are associated with the arousal response, a sudden change in the depth of the sleep during which the individual either arrives in the lighter sleep stage or actually wakes up (**Box 3**). The micro-arousals are short lasting, with periods of bruxism lasting 3 to 15 s with cortical activation associated with an increase in the activity of the sympathetic nervous system. This centrally mediated bruxism is often accompanied by increased muscle activity and gross body movements including involuntary leg movements, increased heart rate, and respiratory changes.

Bruxism should not be considered a pathologic condition and is not an indicator of psychopathology and most individuals with bruxism do not develop pain. Unless bruxism is causing headaches, facial pain, TMJ instability, severe tooth attrition, fracture of dental restorations, or tooth mobility, it does not require treatment. When necessary, the focus of therapy is to prevent damage to the teeth and supporting structures by managing the forces, and this can be accomplished with an intraoral appliance (IOA). Injection of botulinum toxin, which acts as a paralytic, into the temporalis and masseter muscles has been used in patients with cerebral palsy to reduce intraoral soft-tissue injury and tooth damage as well as for patients with bruxism-related headaches. However, the effect of this neurotoxin is localized at the motor

Table 2
Causes of TMD

Cause	Examples	Predisposing	Precipitating	Perpetuating
Trauma, micro	Repetitive strain (eg, wind musician, violin, singing, fingernail biting, scuba diving, snorkeling, swimming)	✓	✓	✓
Trauma, macro	External blow (eg, falls, motor vehicle accident, sports injury, physical abuse, intubation, tooth extraction, prolonged mouth opening, cervical traction, neck brace)		✓	
Ligament laxity, systemic (hypermobility)	Hormonal variation in ligament laxity, Breighton syndrome	✓		✓
Stress-induced parafunction	Tooth clenching, grinding, tapping	✓	✓	✓
Sleep-induced bruxism	Involuntary nocturnal tooth grinding	✓	✓	✓
Restrictive anterior bite relationship	Deep overbite, retruded upper incisors, mandibular skeletal hyperplasia	✓		✓
Loss of posterior tooth support	Missing or extracted molars without prosthetic replacement	✓	✓	✓
Excessive horizontal overjet	>6-mm distance between upper and lower incisors	✓	✓	✓
Abnormal condylar form, developmental or congenital	Bifid condyle, condylar hyperplasia, condylar hypoplasias, tumors	✓		✓
Systemic inflammatory and metabolic polyarthritis	Rheumatoid arthritis, juvenile idiopathic arthritis, scleroderma, psoriatic arthritis, ankylosing spondylitis, Reiter syndrome, systemic lupus erythematosus, gout	✓	✓	✓
Infectious arthritis	Lyme disease, sexually transmitted disease, gonococcal arthritis, Chlamydia trachomatis		✓	
Central nervous system–mediated maxillofacial movement disorders and palsy	Hypokinesia (eg, Parkinson disease, muscular dystrophy), hyperkinesias (eg, tics, tardive dyskinesia, dystonia, chorea, myoclonus), palsy (cerebral palsy, facial palsy)	✓		✓

Box 2
Bruxism (tooth clenching and grinding): reducing bruxism-related symptoms

What are the signs and symptoms of bruxism?

Bruxism activity while you are asleep, especially tooth grinding, occurs more often if you experience restless sleep. Tooth grinding during your sleep is triggered by impulses from the brain and it is not really a habit.

Daytime bruxism is more likely to manifest as tooth clenching or bracing your jaw with your mouth part-way open or off to the side.

Bruxism often leads to tooth sensitivity to hot and cold and to bite pressure.

Cracks in your teeth or flat spots (facets) are another sign of bruxism.

Awakening with a headache or unexplained earache accompanied by a stiff jaw strongly suggests nighttime bruxism.

What should you do if your clench or grind your teeth?

Sleep-related bruxism can be hard to control. You can focus on preventing damage to your teeth and reduce the associated muscle discomfort by using a protective plastic guard over your teeth.

To control daytime clenching or bracing, you have to become aware of the activity. Have those around you remind you if they see your jaw set tight. When you catch yourself clenching remember to keep your lips together and teeth apart.

Consider attending relaxation therapy, biofeedback, or yoga classes to help reduce stress. Increase your physical exercise to improve your sleep.

Avoid excessive caffeine intake or drinking caffeinated beverages within 3 hours of bedtime. Be aware that chocolate and many soda drinks contain caffeine.

Create a quiet and dark sleep environment and establish a regular bedtime. Do not shortchange yourself on sleep.

---

endplate and although the amount of force generated is reduced, it does not alter the bruxism activity and is effective for only 3 to 4 months. Bruxism can also be reduced with the use of sedative and anxiolytic drugs, but patient compliance is low because of side effects. Maintenance of the drugs' therapeutic efficacy, their long-term tolerability, and the risk of addiction need further investigation. Pharmacologic management of bruxism in children is not an appropriate treatment, except for short-term use for situational anxiety. No effective treatment to permanently eliminate sleep bruxism has been identified.

Malocclusion

The clear lack of an association between occlusal anomalies and TMD may be due to the frequent deviation from the norm and because inadequate and invalid study designs, including the failure to take into account the development stage of the occlusion, have led to false-negative results. A sample of 4724 children (2353 girls and 2371 boys) aged 5 to 17 years were grouped by the stage of dental development (deciduous, early mixed, late mixed, and permanent dentition).[37] The registrations included functional occlusion (anterior and lateral sliding, interferences), dental wear, mandibular mobility (maximal opening, deflection), and TMJ and muscular pain provoked by palpation. Mild clinical signs were recorded in 22.8% of the children; only 2.8% had moderate to severe findings and multiple clinical signs. The prevalence of TMD increased during the developmental stages, with girls more affected than boys.

Box 3
Sleep hygiene

Restless or disturbed sleep usually increases bruxism (tooth clenching or grinding). A good night's sleep can be achieved by following these simple guidelines:

Go to bed at about the same time every night and get up from bed at about the same time each day; by doing so the body clock remains synchronized with the outside environment. Everyone has a circadian rhythm, an internal 24-hour clock that plays a critical role in when we fall asleep and when we wake up. By sticking to a regular waking and sleeping time, the body becomes adapted to this schedule.

Exercise regularly. Studies have shown that regular exercise encourages restful sleep. Exercise should be done early in the evening or in the morning. Do not exercise just before bedtime as this stimulates the body and makes it more difficult to fall sleep. Make the bedroom as restful as possible by keeping the temperature cool and reducing noise and outside light to a minimum.

Caffeine is a central nervous system stimulant, temporarily warding off drowsiness and restoring alertness. Avoid chocolate and beverages containing caffeine, such as coffee, tea, soft drinks, and energy drinks for at least 4 hours before bedtime. Do not use alcohol to help you sleep as alcohol consumption leads to fragmented sleep and it often worsens snoring and sleep apnea.

Do not undertake stimulating activities just before bed. Exciting games or movies or engaging in important family discussions stimulate the mind and may make it more difficult to fall asleep.

A warm bath or shower before bedtime increases body temperature and the subsequent decrease in temperature promotes sleep.

If unable to fall asleep within 20 to 30 minutes, get up and engage in some activity in another room. Do not stay in the bedroom trying to force yourself to fall sleep. Only return to the bedroom when you are sleepy.

Significant associations were found between TMD and posterior crossbite, anterior openbite, Angle Class III malocclusion, and extreme maxillary overjet greater than 6 mm.

The occurrence of occlusal anomalies is similar for both sexes, so occlusal factors do not explain the predominance of TMD pain among girls. Although the role of occlusion as a predisposing factor cannot be confirmed by conclusive scientific evidence, some occlusal features may place greater adaptive demands on the masticatory system. It is proposed that most individuals compensate without problems, but adaptation in others may lead to greater risk of dysfunction. Some occlusal anomalies may be a result rather than a cause of TMD.[38]

The relationship between dental occlusion and TMDs has been one of the most controversial topics in the dental community. The Study of Health in Pomerania (Germany), a cross-sectional survey of 4289 adults (aged 20–81 years), revealed associations between 15 occlusion-related variables and TMD signs or symptoms. However, statistical associations do not prove causality. Only bruxism, loss of posterior support, and unilateral posterior crossbite show some consistency across studies. On the other hand, several reported occlusal features seem to be a consequence of TMDs, not their cause. Biological plausibility for the cause of occlusion is often difficult to establish, because TMDs are much more common among women than men. Symptom improvement after insertion of an IOA or after occlusal adjustment does not prove an occlusal cause, because the amelioration may be the result of appliance-induced changes in vertical dimension, or altered proprioception with decreased muscle activity. In addition, TMD symptoms often abate even in the absence of therapy.[39]

Systemic Factors

Most connective tissue diseases that affect other articulations also occur in the TMJ, including rheumatoid arthritis, ankylosing spondylitis, systemic lupus erythematosus, mixed connective tissue disease, juvenile idiopathic arthritis, and psoriatic arthropathy. Typical imaging findings are joint-space narrowing, and condylar erosion, flattening, and sclerosis. Connective tissue diseases are a group of closely related conditions, with many overlapping clinical features that involve the skin, joints, muscles, or blood. Serologic examination can reveal connective tissue diseases that are associated with a variety of antinuclear antigens (ANA) and other related antibodies. However, the ANA test lacks specificity and the presence of the antibody is not necessarily diagnostic for a specific disease because these antibodies may be found in patients with other autoimmune diseases such as hepatitis C, may be induced by medication, and may even be present in otherwise healthy individuals.

Generalized joint hypermobility (GJH) was evaluated as a risk factor for TMD in 895 subjects (20–60 years of age). Hypermobile subjects had a higher risk for reproducible reciprocal TMJ clicking associated with disk displacement with reduction (odds ratio [OR] = 1.68) compared with those without hypermobile joints. No association was observed between hypermobility and myalgia/arthralgia; thus, GJH was found to be associated with nonpainful subtypes of TMD.[40]

Children (n = 1833) aged 4 to 18 years were evaluated for GJH; the prevalence rate of symptomatic hypermobility was 13.8% for girls and 8.2% for boys. Besides gender (OR = 2.07), risk factors for symptomatic hypermobility were race (OR = 2.61 for nonwhites) and was associated with masticatory muscle pain (OR = 1.95).[41]

Trauma

In a survey of 2374 students, 715 had positive symptoms for TMD. They were classified into 7 groups: group 1, those with clicking only; group 2, only pain in the temporomandibular joint; group 3, only difficulty with mouth opening; group 4, clicking and pain; group 5, clicking and difficulty with mouth opening; group 6, difficulty with mouth opening and pain; and group 7, all 3 symptoms. TMD symptoms were significantly associated with a history of jaw injury with; the ORs by group were: group 2, 2.25; group 3, 2.47; group 6, 3.38; and group 7, 2.01. Experience of third molar removal was significantly associated with the onset of TMD (OR = 1.81) for group 1. Experiences of jaw injury and third molar removal might be cumulative and precipitating events in TMD. No association was found between orthodontic experience and TMD in any group.[42]

The epidemiology of facial injuries in children and adolescents (from birth to 18 years) was evaluated using the National Trauma Data Bank (2001–2005) to examine facial fracture pattern, mechanism, and concomitant injury by age. A total of 12,739 (4.6%) facial fractures were identified among 277,008 pediatric trauma patient admissions. The proportion of patients with facial fractures increased substantially with age. The most common facial fractures were mandible (32.7%), nasal (30.2%), and maxillary/zygoma (28.6%). Motor vehicle collision (55.1%), assault (14.5%), and falls (8.6%) were the most common mechanisms for facial fracture in all pediatric age groups. The second most common cause of bony facial injury varied with age. Fall was the second most common mechanism (23.4%) among infants and toddlers (0–4 years). Bicycle-related collisions and pedestrians struck by motor vehicles were the second most common mechanisms for school-aged children (5–14 years). For older teenagers (15–18 years), the second most common mechanism was a fight or an assault (21.7%). The male sex predominated through all age groups and for all types of injuries.[43]

Related to increasing age, many of these patients reported more than one trauma, and as pointed out by Akhter and colleagues,[42] there is a cumulative effect of trauma as a causative factor for TMD. Of the in 644 children (**Fig. 3**) seeking TMD treatment, 13.8% presented with chin scars and 37.7% reported a history of facial trauma that may have contributed to their TMD. Although not statistically significant, because of the small number of males in the sample, blows to the face are more common in males.

EXAMINATION FOR TMDS
Range of Motion

Mandibular range of motion (ROM) assessment is a simple and objective method to evaluate the function of the masticatory system and both reduced and excessive mandibular mobility can be seen in TMD. Mandibular ROM is directly related to height. The ability of the patient to place 3 fingers vertically in a handshake position between the incisor teeth (the 3-finger test) approximates a normal range of mandibular opening of 35 to 50 mm.[44] If it is not possible to get even 2 fingers between the patient's incisal edges, then the reason for the limited opening should be investigated. Excursive mandibular movement to each side is normally 8 to 10 mm. The width of a permanent maxillary central incisor is 8 to 9 mm, so if the patient can move the lower jaw sideways by the width of an upper central incisor, this should be considered normal. Pain, mandibular deviation, end-point deflection, catching, or locking associated with these movements should be noted.

Provocation of Masticatory Muscle Pain

Firm bilateral pressure applied to the temporalis and masseter muscles while the patient is clenching will reveal tenderness and determine if there is atrophy or hypertrophy, which may be associated with extreme bruxism.

Temporomandibular Joint Palpation and Load Testing

The lateral aspect of the capsule of the TMJ is examined by having the patient open their mouth halfway while the clinician firmly presses the index fingers in the depression created behind each condyle, just in front of the tragus of the ear. The presence of discomfort is noted as the patient slowly opens and closes. With the mouth half open, the patient should move the mandible from side to side. Joint loading is accomplished by the clinician applying force under the angle of the mandible, with the teeth slightly out of contact. Functional loading while chewing on a cotton roll or wax between the last molars provides information about contralateral capsular pain. This squeezing action torques the TMJ on the opposite side and can trigger the clicking and the joint or muscle pain that the patient experiences while chewing. Biting on tongue blades on the side of joint pain may reduce the pain if it is related to inflammation. TMJ palpation also allows the clinician to feel asynchronous or irregular movements and clicking or crepitation.

Differentiation of TMJ Sounds

TMJ sounds are categorized as

- Clicking (popping and snapping)
- Soft-tissue crepitus
- Hard-tissue grating

A stethoscope applied lightly over the joint is helpful in distinguishing the character and intensity of sounds. The noise should be evaluated on opening, closing, and in excursive jaw movements. Applying upward pressure at the angle of the mandible usually increases the intensity of the sound and this should be done if the patient reports a recent history of sounds but none were detected in unloaded jaw movements.

The most common cause of TMJ sounds is disc displacement or internal derangement, but altered synovial lubrication, intracapsular adhesions, deviations in the shape of the disc, condyle, or tubercle, and incoordination between the disc and condyle during movement can all cause TMJ sounds.

Not all TMJ internal derangements are progressive, and clicking might not change in character over time. TMJ noise can diminish in frequency and intensity without any intervention. The resolution of joint sounds does not always equate with the absence of a pathologic condition. When a displaced disc becomes nonreducing, known as a closed-lock of the TMJ, the condyle no longer translates onto the displaced disc and there is cessation of joint sounds with associated limitation of ROM and deflection on opening to the affected side.

TMJ IMAGING

When the clinician is faced with numerous and conflicting concepts of TMD etiology and when there is diagnostic uncertainty, the patients may be being subjected to costly, unnecessary, and unproved ancillary diagnostic procedures to evaluate TMJ sounds, altered ROM, and facial pain. Imaging of TMJ is recommended when there is a recent history of mandibular trauma, evidence of developing facial asymmetry, or when hard-tissue grinding or crepitus is detected, but it should not be considered a routine part of the diagnostic evaluation.

Mandibular condyles are subject to significant changes in size and shape during childhood growth. As the size of the condyles increases, the angle decreases and therefore the position of the condyle within the fossa changes. The shape of the mandibular condyles turns from a round into an oval configuration.[45] These age-related changes of the mandibular condyle need to be taken into consideration when imaging the TMJ in children.

Imaging of the TMJ is most commonly accomplished with a panoramic view because of its relatively low cost, widespread availability, and minimal radiation. Panoramic images of the TMJ are reliable for evaluating condylar head morphology and angulation and cortex density but do not permit evaluation of joint space or condylar motion. Panoramic images are useful for measuring vertical ramus height, which has been shown to be reduced in growing children with disc displacement.[46] A steeper mandibular plane angle, increased antegonial notching, and skeletal facial asymmetry, all visualized on a panoramic image, are seen more often in patients with TMD.[47]

Computed tomography (CT) or cone beam computed tomography (CBCT) volumetric imaging is indicated for the detection of TMJ osseous abnormalities, fracture detection, and analysis of facial asymmetry, but results in considerably more radiation exposure than panoramic imaging and their use should be selective. Magnetic resonance imaging (MRI) produces no ionizing radiation and provides visualization of the position and contours of the TMJ disc and other soft tissues, can detect inflammation, and often improves diagnostic accuracy.

Subchondral formation of cortical bone in the condyles of adolescents and young adults was evaluated with CBCT in 1438 patients between 10 and 30 years of age. No patient had signs or symptoms of TMD. Subchondral formation of cortical bone was first seen at the age of 13 to 14 years in boys and 12 to 13 years in girls. The cortical bone begins to form around the periphery of the condyles during adolescence (12–14 years). A continuous, homogeneous, and compact cortical bony layer is established in young adults by the age of 22 years for men and 21 for women, indicating full development of the mandibular condyle.[48] This documentation of the cessation of active growth in the condylar region has implications for the timing of both orthodontic treatment and orthognathic surgical treatment.

TMJ BIOMECHANICS

The interposed disc functions as a shock absorber and serves as a congruous surface between the incongruous condyle and articular tubercle. The complex hinge and sliding movements of the compound TMJ are facilitated by the independent rotation and translation of the disc over the condylar head. This shifting position of the disc acts as a moving wedge that maintains near-continuous contact between the disc-condyle complex and the articular tubercle during chewing.

When the mouth is opened, the initial movement is primarily the condylar head rotating against the inferior surface of the stationary disc. As the degree of opening increases, the disc rotates posteriorly on the condyle and together the disc-condyle complex translates forward and downward, guided by contact of the disc's upper surface against the inclined articular tubercle. With wide opening, the condyle and disc translate smoothly together to the edge of or beyond the apex of the articular tubercle (**Fig. 5**).

CLINICAL FINDINGS IN TMDS

The three cardinal features of TMDs are orofacial pain, jaw joint noises, and restricted jaw function. The symptoms are often remitting but recurring, and can continue long

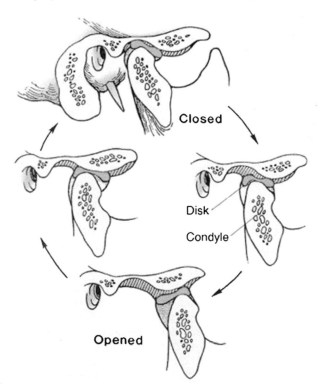

Fig. 5. Normal relationship of the disc and condyle during the mouth opening and closing cycle. Translation of the disc and condyle to or just beyond the height of the tubercle is a normal finding.

after the precipitating event. Thus, identifying and managing perpetuating factors may be even more important than determining the predisposing and precipitating factors.

Parker[49] outlined a dynamic model of TMDs with a shifting balance between adaptation and dysfunction. This model helps explain the multiple variations in the clinical presentation of TMD and why a variety of treatment modalities promote homeostasis and result in symptomatic relief, even when the underlying causes have not been identified. Clark[50] advocated a multifactorial model of TMD causation and clarified how dentistry's historical mechanical emphasis on malocclusion and abnormal structure of the jaws ignored biological diversity and adaptability. Clark stressed that the anatomic susceptibility of TMJ articular tissues to trauma, polyarthritic diseases, joint laxity, repetitive parafunctional behaviors, and stress-related muscle dysfunction all need to be recognized and treated.

Habits

Fingernail biting is a surprisingly common habit, and examination of fingernails and cuticles should be included in a TMJ screening examination. A questionnaire completed by 2905 students revealed a declining prevalence of fingernail biting with age. Nail-biting was acknowledged by 28% of students aged 15 to 19 years and by 21% of college students aged 21 to 26 years.[51] In a study of 1077 college students, 29.3% of men and 19.3% of women were active nail-biters. Social disapproval of nail-biting could have more impact on women, thus explaining the sex difference. Compared with controls, nail-biters have higher anxiety scores. Experimental studies have shown that the repetitive mandibular protrusion, necessary for fingernail biting, creates preauricular pain from lateral pterygoid muscle fatigue. The TMJ is loaded more heavily when biting with the incisors, as in fingernail biting, than when biting an object between the molar teeth.[52]

A simple and effective treatment of nail-biting is to have the patient place a small adhesive bandage over the fingernail on 1 finger the first week, 2 fingernails the second week, 3 fingernails the third week, and continue to increase the number of fingernails covered by bandages each week. Given motivation from the knowledge that this habit is contributing to facial pain, this simple behavior modifier often enables the patient to stop nail-biting within a few weeks.

Biting of objects such as pens, pencils, paperclips, hairpins, split ends of hair, or other objects should be investigated, and lip, cheek, and tongue biting can be noted by careful observation while taking the oral history and by examining the intraoral soft tissues for mucosal ridging or irritation. Pereira and colleagues[5] found that there is not a significant correlation between oral habits, such as pacifier sucking, nonnutritive sucking, finger sucking and nail-biting, and signs and symptoms of TMD.

Juvenile Idiopathic Arthritis

Juvenile idiopathic arthritis (JIA) is defined as persistent arthritis for more than 6 weeks with an onset at younger than 16 years of age, after excluding other causes of joint inflammation. JIA is the most common autoimmune autoinflammatory musculoskeletal disease in childhood. Involvement of the TMJ is common and children with JIA present a remarkable prevalence of condylar destruction, yet they are often asymptomatic and thus overlooked. The presence of anterior openbite and antegonial notching and shortened posterior ramal height of the mandible with retroganthia are all important clues (**Fig. 6**). With panoramic imaging in patients with the polyarticular type of JIA, 75% of the children have radiographic changes of the condyles and 55.6% have bilateral lesions. The TMJ can be affected early or late in the course of the disease, and can even be the first joint involved.[53] Larheim and Rönning[54] imaged

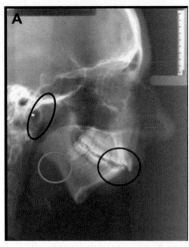
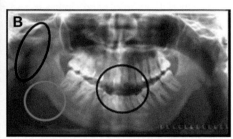

Fig. 6. Lateral (*A*) and cephalometric (*B*) images of a 15-year-old boy with JIA demonstrating condylar resorption (blue), antegonial notching (green), and anterior dental openbite (red).

85 patients with JIA with orthopantomogram and lateral cephalograms and reported that if the condyles were affected, 82% had retrognathia and 58% had posterior rotation of the mandible. The clinician should be concerned about JIA if panoramic imaging reveals the triad of condylar resorption, antegonial notching, and anterior dental openbite (see **Fig. 6**).

Abnormal Tooth Wear

Dental erosion, the dissolution of hard tooth tissues caused by acids of nonbacterial origin, can cause extreme loss of tooth material, especially if combined with mechanical factors in the mouth. The best approach to prevent the problem is to reduce the acid challenges in the mouth. This, however, poses a problem when dealing with erosion caused by intrinsic factors such as gastrointestinal problems or low patient compliance in erosion caused by an acidic diet.

Abrasion caused by tooth grinding may be related to SB, classified as a parasomnia, a group of sleep disturbances that also includes sleep walking, nightmares, sleep talking, and enuresis[55] Bruxism can also occur in association with medications used for mood and anxiety disorders, attention-deficit/hyperactivity disorder,[56] and in those with pervasive developmental disorders and autism spectrum disorder.[57]

Erosion of the lingual surfaces of the upper teeth caused by the regurgitation of stomach acids associated with bulimia is easily detected. Bulimia, a cycle of food binges followed by purging, has an estimated incidence of 2.1% in young women; men account for less than 10% of those with bulimia.[58] Up to 60% of patients with bulimia nervosa report previous histories of anorexia nervosa. Severe dental erosion and dental caries were significantly more common among patients with bulimia than controls, as was increased tooth sensitivity to cold and pressure. Eating disorders, TMD, and chronic facial pain coexist, and in the eating disorder population, 60.9% report facial pain currently or in the recent past. Both conditions often have an underlying psychological component to their origin and are associated with other psychological comorbidities. The parotid salivary secretory patterns in 28 patients with bulimia were determined to investigate functional abnormality in the glands.[59] Patients with bulimia had a reduced resting flow rate, and salivary amylase activity was increased in both resting and stimulated states. Bilateral parotid gland enlargement was observed in 25% of patients with bulimia nervosa. Ultrasonography of 45 females with eating disorders and 25 controls between 16 and 40 years of age revealed the parotid gland was more than twice as large in those with bulimia that those in the control group. Submandibular glands were not enlarged. Videofluorography of the pharynx, larynx, and esophagus of 13 patients with bulimia compared with 13 age-matched controls revealed the pharyngeal gag reflex was absent in 9 of the 13 patients with bulimia and only 1 patient had a velar gag reflex. All 13 controls had both gag reflexes.[60] A diminished gag reflex results from the hand or other object being repetitively placed down the throat to induce vomiting, and skin abrasions, lacerations, and calluses, called Russell's sign, may be present on the dorsum of the hands, caused by contact with the teeth when attempting to stimulate regurgitation. Repetitive vomiting can result in TMJ hyperextension and sprain. Headaches can occur as a result of the poor nutritional status and from the strain imposed on the temporalis muscles from TMJ hypermobility.

Internal Derangements

If an internal derangement develops,[61] the disc usually displaces anteromedially in the direction of the pterygoid plate, the origin of the lateral pterygoid. However, depending on the stage of the internal derangement, bony anatomy, and the specific cause of the disc displacement, a variety of other disc positions, including partial disc displacement, have been identified with MRI. TMJ clicking occurs when the condyle travels over the band of the displaced disc, and the sound occurs as the condyle impacts against the temporal bone through the thin central portion of the disc (**Fig. 7**).

The initial stage of a TMJ internal derangement is characterized by clicking on opening, closing, and in translation. Progressive disc displacement and deformation of the disc can change the character, position, and intensity of TMJ sounds. If the posterior band of the displaced disc becomes thinner over time, the clicking diminishes. If instead the posterior band becomes thicker, and if the attachments of the disc become further stretched, episodes of catching and locking can occur. If the disc bunches up in front of the condyle, the condylar translation and mouth opening will be limited (**Fig. 8**).

On average, 70% of mouth opening is achieved by condylar rotation, so even when there is a disc displacement that blocks translation, the patient can usually open about 30 mm. With progression to a nonreducing disc displacement, there is often an increase in joint pain because of the additional strain placed on the highly vascularized and innervated retrodiscal tissue. Progressive thinning of the posterior attachment or retrodiscal tissue can result in a perforation and the onset of crepitus. Nonreducing displacements are often accompanied by alterations in condylar position and morphology, and can result in discernible changes in the bite.

Joint Hypermobility

In some instances, the condyle subluxates beyond the anterior band of the disc (**Fig. 9**), which can result in episodes of painful jaw-locking in an open position. The hypermobile TMJ ROM typically exceeds 60 mm, with the click usually occurring at greater than 30 mm of opening. With TMJ subluxation, the closing click is often louder than the opening click. In contrast, TMJ clicking caused by disc displacement usually occurs at less than 30 mm of opening, and the opening click is louder than the closing click.

Subluxations or dislocations are displacement of the head of the condyle out of the glenoid fossa and are influenced by the morphology of the condyle, glenoid fossa, and

INTERNAL DERANGEMENTS

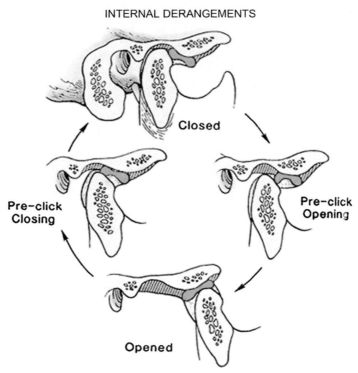

Fig. 7. Temporomandibular joint clicking associated with a displaced disc. The click on opening occurs as the condyle and disc realign and is usually louder than the closing click, which occurs as the disc again displaces as the mouth is closed.

articular eminence. A steepening of the slope of the eminence takes place in 3 phases, paralleling the eruption of the central incisors, the permanent first molars, and the permanent second molars.[62] The inclination of the articular eminence changes rapidly until the completion of deciduous dentition, attaining more or less 45% of its adult value. By the age of 10 years, it is 70% to 72% completed, and by the age of 20 years, it is 90% to 94% completed.[63] Thus, young children can make exaggerated jaw movements involving translation of the condyle past the height of the eminence, but the slope of the eminence is so flat that they can easily reposition their condyle without any catching or locking. The same degree of translation associated with opening after the age of complete eruption of their dentition and development of a steeper articular eminence is more likely to be problematic.

Open jaw-locking is usually secondary to an interruption in the normal sequence of muscle action when attempting to close the mouth from extreme opening.[64] The masseter and temporalis muscles elevate the mandible before the lateral pterygoid muscle relaxes, resulting in the mandibular condyle being pulled out of the glenoid fossa and anterior to the bony eminence (**Fig. 10**). Spasm of the masseter, temporalis, and pterygoid muscles causes trismus and keeps the condyle from returning into the glenoid fossa. The frequency of recurrent subluxation or dislocation and self-reducibility can be inversely linked to the height of the articular eminence. Predisposing factors in children include epilepsy, vomiting including that associated with bulimia, Ehlers-Danlos syndrome, Marfan syndrome and system ligament laxity, and dystonic

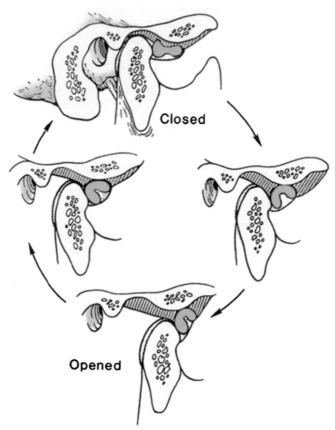

Fig. 8. Anteromedial disc displacement without reduction (nonreducing disc displacement). The condyle engages the posterior aspect of the deformed and displaced disc on opening or in protrusion, blocking the translation of the condyle.

movements from the effect of major tranquilizers/neuroleptics used for neuropsychiatric diseases.[65]

TREATMENT

A 14-year-old girl experienced repetitive subluxations and presented with excessive mandibular ROM of 63 mm (see **Fig. 10**). After repeated manual reduction in an emergency room, she was placed on a liquid diet and provided with a bandage warp (**Fig. 11**), which was being worn 24 hours a day. A CBCT image revealed normal condylar and eminence morphology and excessive condylar translation (**Fig. 12**). Bonded lingual buttons were placed on the facial surface of the 4 canine teeth so that the patient can wear interarch elastic bands or closing chains on both sides of the mouth (**Fig. 13**). The elastic restraints limit the opening about to 25 mm, thus allowing near full rotation but limiting translation. Before bedtime, a shorter elastic chain is applied to limit lateral excursive movements that occur from pressure on the mandible related to sleep posture. The use of this temporary restraint promotes cautious eating habits and controls unexpected yawns. The elastics do not cause eruption of the canine teeth and are not uncomfortable to wear.

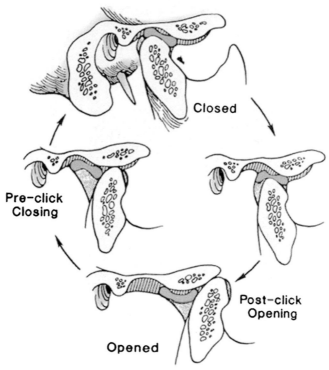

Closed

Pre-click
Closing

Post-click
Opening

Opened

Fig. 9. Condylar hypermobility with clicking occurring on wide opening as the condyle translates beyond the height of the tubercle and over the anterior band of the disc. The clicking on closing is usually louder than the opening click and occurs as the disc recenters over the condyle on mouth closure.

Prolonged thumb-sucking, which has contributed to an anterior openbite (**Fig. 13**), may be a cofactor in the cause of her subluxation problem, but both she and her mother have systemic ligament laxity; both can bend their thumb to their forearm (**Fig. 14**).

Dozens of similar cases of repetitive dislocation/subluxation have been successfully treated in vocalists, those with bulimia, and those with seizure disorders or medication side effects. The elastic restraint is continued for 8 to 12 months; the overall success rate is lower in those patients who have systemic ligament laxity. These patients are

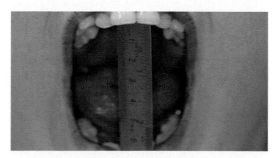

Fig. 10. Fourteen-year-old girl with 63-mm mouth opening between incisal edges.

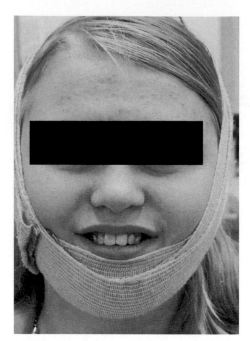

Fig. 11. Restraint used by patient to prevent repetitive open-mouth locking episodes.

also instructed in a hinge axis jaw exercise to maximize condylar rotations and minimize translation. IOA therapy is used in conjunction with the elastic restraint only if there is a need to control forces related to bruxism. Eminectomy to prevent condylar locking by improving the ease of closing or zygomatic down-fracture to prevent condylar translation both act on the bony obstacle, but do not have a therapeutic effect on TMJ ligament and capsular laxity or masticatory muscle activity.

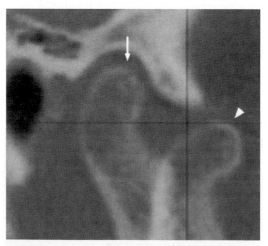

Fig. 12. Superimposition of the right TMJ condylar position with teeth together (*arrow*) beyond the tubercle associated with open-mouth locking (*triangle*).

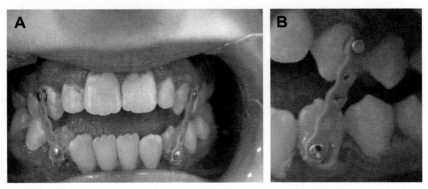

Fig. 13. (*A, B*) Bonded orthodontic lingual buttons and removable elastic chains to limit mouth opening to 25 mm.

Even when a specific TMD diagnosis is established, the clinician may be reluctant to recommend therapy because clear criteria have not been established for selection of the diverse treatments advocated for TMJ dysfunction.[66] A study of 145 patients with TMD randomly referred to 2 clinics revealed that despite the markedly different diagnostic and treatment methods used, there were no important differences in treatment outcomes at 1-year follow-up.[67] This variability in clinical methods for treating TMD, especially the use of irreversible and surgical therapy, is not a benign phenomenon.

The efficacy of IOAs for managing TMD in adults is documented,[68] but there is a lack of understanding of why appliances are effective.[69] Successful appliance therapy for TMD has been attributed to: (1) modifying the occlusal relationship, (2) managing the forces associated with bruxism, (3) altering the zone of loading on the TMJ.[70] An IOA should not be used in isolation and should be considered as an adjunct to selfcare, physiotherapy, and, when appropriate, antiinflammatory medications and sleep aides.

The efficacy of IOA treatment in children is less certain and there no clear evidence-based protocol for using appliances in children. Appliance therapy for TMD in children in primary or mixed dentition is a more complicated task than for adults. Primary teeth lack the retention of the permanent dentition and the process of exfoliation and eruption makes the fitting of and the ongoing adjustment of these appliances a challenge. The level of compliance with appliance use is often more of a problem than it is with

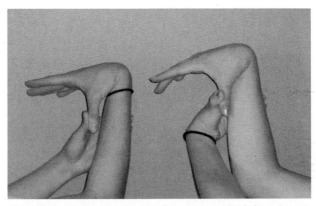

Fig. 14. Hyperextensibility of thumb to wrist of patient on the left and mother on the right.

TMJ Disorder Examination

RANGE OF MOTION:

		Pain	
		Joint	Muscle
Active mandibular opening	___mm	NO R L	R L
Passive assisted opening	___mm	NO R L	R L
Protrusive opening passive (POM)	___mm	NO R L	R L
End-point deflection on opening to the NO R L			
Right lateral movement	___mm	NO R L	R L
Left lateral movement	___mm	NO R L	R L
Protrusive movement	___mm	NO R L	R L

TMJ TENDERNESS: **PAIN**
Lateral palpation - static - closed   NO   R   L
Lateral palpation - dynamic – open and side-to-side   NO   R   L
Static joint loading causes pain (bimanual)   NO   R   L
                                                          SOUNDS
Dynamic loading causes pain- right side chewing   NO   R   L   NO   R L
                      - left side chewing   NO   R   L   NO   R   L

MUSCLE TENDERNESS:
Temporalis – anterior   0 1 2 3   0 1 2 3
Superficial masseter   0 1 2 3   0 1 2 3
Deep masseter   0 1 2 3   0 1 2 3

JOINT SOUNDS:
Click and Popping   NO ___mm   NO ___mm
Crepitus/Grating   NO ___mm   NO ___mm
Click/Pop in protrusive excursion   NO R L
Click/Pop reduced if opening from edge to edge   NO R L
Crepitus/Grating increased if opening from edge to edge   NO R L

OCCLUSAL FINDINGS:
Vertical Overbite ___mm or ___%   Horizontal Overjet ___mm
Angle's Classification   R 1 2 3   L 1 2 3   Div I II

Midlines   Crossbite NO R L Ant   Open bite NO R L Ant

Abnormal tooth wear   Anterior 0 1 2 3   Canines 0 1 2 3   Posterior 0 1 2 3
                           Evidence of erosion   Y N   GERD suspected   Y N
Anterior tooth mobility __ __ __ __ __ __   Anterior Fremitus __ __ __ __ __ __
Ridging of buccal mucosa Y N   Tongue scalloped Y N   Tongue thrust Y N

FACIAL SYMMETRY
Chin scar   Y N   History of mandibular trauma _____
Maxillary asymmetry N R L   Mandibular asymmetry   N R L
Ligament laxity of thumb to wrist Y N
Fingernail Biting   Y N
Comments_____

Fig. 15. TMJ disorder examination form.

adults. These complications, coupled with the minimal training of most pediatric dentists in managing TMD and bruxism, can result in the clinician being dismissive of questions raised by the patient or parent regarding TMDs and bruxism.

All IOA designs have the potential to

1. Alter the occlusal condition
2. Alter the condylar position
3. Increase the vertical dimension
4. Create cognitive awareness

TMJ Disorder History

Do you experience jaw fatigue or pain?   F S N
   If there is jaw pain, does it occur when the jaw is
       [ ] stationary or at rest
       [ ] with chewing or speaking
       [ ] upon wide opening/yawning/singing

| F = Frequently |
| S = Sometimes |
| N = Never |

Do you have jaw/ear/facial pain upon awakening, prior to jaw use?
                                      Right side   F S N
                                      Left side   F S N

Do you have headaches upon awakening?   F S N

Has a physician advised you that that you have migraine headaches?   Y N

Do you have limitation of mouth opening?   F S N
   If so, was the onset   [ ] gradual   [ ] sudden
   Is the limitation present upon awakening?   F S N

Is there jaw joint clicking or popping?   Right side   F S N
                                        Left side   F S N

Is there jaw joint crepitus or a hard tissue grating?   Right side   F S N
                                        Left side   F S N

Is there jaw   Right side   [ ] catching   [ ] locking?   F S N
          Left side   [ ] catching   [ ] locking?   F S N
  If so, does this occur   [ ] with chewing   [ ] with yawning   [ ] during/after dental visits

Are you aware of a recent change in your bite or the way your teeth fit together?   Y N

Is there a history of a fall or other trauma to the face or lower jaw?   Y N

Have you had any recent images or x-rays of your head or jaws, including CTs or MRIs that may
have been taken for sinus problem or headaches?_____ Y N

Have you played any wind instruments or the violin or viola?   Y N
   If yes, Years_____ Which instruments(s)? _____

Have you received orthodontic treatment? Years_____ Dr. _____ Y N

Do you suspect tooth [ ] clenching [ ] grinding suspected? [ ] Not aware of clenching or grinding
Do you have difficulty falling asleep?   F S N
Do you have restless sleep?   F S N
Are you excessively sleepy or fatigued during the day?   F S N
Do you feel unhappy or depressed?   F S N
Do you become easily upset or irritated?   F S N
Do you consider yourself to be a nervous or anxious person?   F S N
On average, how long does it take you to fall asleep at bedtime?   _____minutes
On average, how many total hours do you sleep each night?   _____hours
Have you been diagnosed with gastro-esophageal reflux disease (GERD)?   Y N

What medications do you take for you jaw pain, earaches and headaches: _____
_____

Comments:_____
_____

Fig. 16. TMJ disorder history form.

Combining magnetic resonance images with jaw tracking (dynamic stereometry), the intraarticular distances of 20 human TMJs before and after insertion of a 3-mm-thick IOA in the first molar region were evaluated. For habitual closure, protrusion, and laterotrusion in the contralateral joint, IOAs led to minor, yet statistically significant increases in the global TMJ space and to larger increases in defined condylar areas. Condylar end rotation and translation in the habitual arc of closure were reduced. Hence, the insertion of a 3-mm-thick IOA led to a change in the

Clinician's Guide for Interpreting the TMJ Examination

Can the patient open their mouth the width of three fingers? [Adult opening: F – 47mm M – 52mm. Under the age of 15 years: 35mm.]

If there is limited mouth opening, is there more than a 5mm increase in opening with passive stretch applied to the incisors by the examiner? *(If yes, this suggests protective muscle splinting rather than a nonreducing disc.)*

Is the opening from a protruded position, by translating the mandible first and then rotating open, less than the opening from maximum intercuspation? *(If yes, this suggests an internal derangement with a nonreducing disc limiting the condylar movement.)*

Are the right and left lateral mandibular excursions of near equal range and at least the width of a central incisor? [Average excursion: 8-12mm.] *(If not equal, the limited excursion may be related to a contralateral internal derangement with a nonreducing disc or degenerative joint disease.)*

Are TMJ clicking or popping sounds evident, on which side, at what range of opening, and in which excursive jaw movements? *(TMJ sounds that occur past 35mm and that do no occur in excursions may be related to hypermobility and joint laxity and the use of an intraoral appliance is not likely to alter the clicking.)*

Does opening and closing in an edge to edge position decrease the noise and is this movement comfortable for the patient? *(Consider using an appliance design that allows or encourages the mandible to posture forward.)*

Is hard tissue grating and crepitus evident? *(Suggests progression to arthrosis with bony remodeling and imaging may be indicated. Contraindicates the use of an appliance that postures the jaw forward. The appliance design should incorporate posterior contact, even if there are missing posterior teeth.)*

Does the hard tissue grating diminish by preventing full closure into centric occlusion, i.e. increasing the posterior vertical dimension? *(If so, fabricate thick appliance (test with tongue blades or wax) to position the condyle away from (decompress) the perforated intracapsular soft tissue.)*

Does opening and closing in an edge to edge position increase the grating noise? *(If so, use an appliance design with anterior guidance that discourages the mandible from posturing forward.)*

Does guiding the jaw open in a retruded, hinge position cause jaw joint pain or locking? *(If so, use appliance design that directs the mandible away from most retruded position, with minimal anterior guidance and with distal occlusal support. Avoid the anterior-only tooth contact or deprogrammer appliance design.)*

Are the masseter and temporalis muscles tender bilaterally or only on the side of a painful TMJ? *(**Bilateral** muscle tenderness is usually associated with bruxism or with bilateral TMJ pain protective muscle splinting. **Unilateral** muscle pain is seldom caused by bruxism and is probably related to reflex protective muscle splinting or guarding a painful TMJ.)*

Is there masseter muscle hypertrophy? *(This finding suggests chronic bruxism. Soft appliances should be avoided as the patient will "work the appliance". Anterior-only contact appliances are contraindicated for patients with masseter hypertrophy because of the amount of force generated on the TMJs when there is no posterior tooth contact.)*

With the patient sitting in an upright position, facing forward, where is the point of initial tooth contact and does this change when the unsupported head is tilted backward? *(When there is unilateral soft tissue or bony deterioration, the mandible often postures in this direction and the initial point of contact will be on the side of the intracapsular change. Unless the tissue adaptation has stopped, it is a mistake to adjust the point of initial tooth contact, as this allows the mandible to posture even more in this direction and may lead to increased loading of the joint.)*

Is there fremitus on the anterior teeth and has the patient noticed a recent change in their bite? *(If the retrodiscal tissues of the TMJ are inflamed or painful, the patient will usually posture the involved jaw joint forward. This can lead to muscle fatigue and also the tell-tale sign of heavy anterior occlusion. With a unilateral jaw problem the heavy contact will usually be on the contralateral anterior teeth. The bite discrepancy may be transient and will no longer be evident when the pain and inflammation resolve.)*

Fig. 17. Interpreting the TMJ examination.

topographic condyle-fossa relationship, and therefore to a new distribution of contact areas between joint surfaces.[71]

Condylar displacement related to the loss of posterior occlusal support was measured in 23 patients with intact dentition who were provided with an IOA covering all teeth. The vertical and horizontal condylar position was measured by an ultrasonic motion analyzer and then the IOA was unilaterally shortened tooth-by-tooth up to the canine tooth and the measurement was repeated after each shortening. Removing the appliance coverage on the second molar on one side lead to a slight ipsilateral cranial condylar motion if the patient clenched with maximum force. When the second and first molars were uncovered, a noticeable cranial condylar movement of about 0.3 mm was observed when the teeth were occluded, even with low force. Long-term wear of anterior-only coverage appliances for bruxism or TMD, especially in a patient with an internal derangement, can alter the occlusion and unfavorably load the TMJ.[72]

TMJ surgery is seldom indicated in growing individuals. There are indications for reconstructive surgery using costochondral grafts.[73] Arthroscopy or arthrocentesis is frequently used in patients with JIA.[74] TMJ ankylosis may require a gap arthroplasty.[75] Most mandibular fractures are treated with closed reductions,[76] but there are indications for open surgical reduction of mandibular fractures with internal fixation.

SUMMARY

The prevalence of TMD in children and adolescents is difficult to establish, but the importance of early detection and appropriate intervention is important to reduce jaw dysfunction and prevent progression. The American Academy of Pediatric Dentistry recommends[77] that every comprehensive dental history and examination (**Fig. 15**) should include a TMJ history and assessment, including questions about mandibular dysfunction (**Fig. 16**) and previous orofacial trauma. In the presence of signs and symptoms of TMD, a more comprehensive examination should include palpation of the masticatory muscles and the TMJs, documentation of joint sounds, occlusal analysis, and assessment of range of mandibular movements (**Fig. 17**).

Mandibular trauma and systemic disease might not directly affect the dentition, but can alter future condylar growth and result in facial asymmetry and skeletal malocclusion. Timely diagnosis can lessen the effect of a TMJ dysfunction or systemic disease on mandibular growth. The absence of guidelines for TMJ in children and adolescents makes it difficult to apply an evidence-based approach, but it is the dentist's responsibility to examine for and classify TMDs and make the decision to observe, treat, or refer.

REFERENCES

1. Howard JA. Temporomandibular joint disorders, facial pain, and dental problems in performing artists. In: Sataloff RT, Brandfonbrener AG, Lederman RJ, editors. Performing arts medicine, chapter 9, 3rd edition. Narberth (PA): Science & Medicine; 2010. p. 151–96.
2. US Census Bureau. Statistical abstract of the United States: 2012. 131st edition. Washington, DC: US Census Bureau; 2011.
3. Barbosa TS, Miyakoda LS, Rocha CP, et al. Temporomandibular disorders and bruxism in childhood and adolescence: review of the literature. Int J Pediatr Otorhinolaryngol 2008;72:299–314.
4. Magnusson T, Egermark I, Carlsson GE. A prospective investigation over two decades of signs and symptoms of temporomandibular disorders and associated variables: a final summary. Acta Odontol Scand 2005;63:99–109.
5. Pereira LJ, Costa RC, Franca JP, et al. Risk indicators for signs and symptoms of temporomandibular dysfunction in children. J Clin Pediatr Dent 2009;34(1):81–6.
6. Nydell A, Helkimo M, Koch G. Craniomandibular disorders in children: a critical review of literature. Swed Dent J 1994;18:191–205.

7. List T, Wahlund K, Wenneberg B, et al. TMD in children and adolescents: prevalence of pain, gender differences, and perceived treatment need. J Orofac Pain 1999;13(1):9–20.

8. Macfarlane TV, Blinkhorn AS, Davies RM, et al. Factors associated with health care seeking behavior for orofacial pain in the general population. Community Dent Health 2003;20(1):20–6.

9. Wahlund K, List T, Dworkin SF. Temporomandibular disorders in children and adolescents: reliability of a questionnaire, clinical examination, and diagnosis. J Orofac Pain 1998;12:42–51.

10. Nilsson IM. Reliability, validity, incidence and impact of temporomandibular pain disorders in adolescents. Swed Dent J Suppl 2007;(183):7–86.

11. Riga M, Xenellis J, Peraki E, et al. Aural symptoms in patients with temporomandibular joint disorders: multiple frequency tympanometry provides objective evidence of changes in middle ear impedance. Otol Neurotol 2010;31(9):1359–64.

12. Cox KW. Temporomandibular disorder and new aural symptoms. Arch Otolaryngol Head Neck Surg 2008;134(4):389–93.

13. Köhler AA, Helkimo A, Magnusson T, et al. Prevalence of symptoms and signs indicative of temporomandibular disorders in children and adolescents. A cross-sectional epidemiological investigation covering two decades. Eur Arch Paediatr Dent 2009;10(Suppl 1):16–25.

14. Dworkin SF, LeResche L. Research diagnostic criteria for temporomandibular disorders: review, criteria, examinations and specifications, critique. J Craniomandib Disord 1992;6:301–55.

15. Palla S. Biopsychosocial pain model crippled? [editorial]. J Orofac Pain 2011; 25(4):290.

16. Klasser GD, Greene CS. The changing field of temporomandibular disorders: what dentists need to know. J Can Dent Assoc 2009;75:49–53.

17. Chambers CT, Craig KD, Bennett SM. The impact of maternal behavior on children's pain experiences: an experimental analysis. J Pediatr Psychol 2002;27: 293–301.

18. Roth-Isigkeit A, Thyen U, Stöven H, et al. Pain among children and adolescents: restrictions in daily living and triggering factors. Pediatrics 2005;15(2):152–62.

19. People statistical notes, no. 20. Atlanta (GA): Centers for Disease Control; 2001.

20. Population estimates. Washington, DC: United States Census Bureau; 2011.

21. Nilsson IM, List T, Drangsholt M. Prevalence of temporomandibular pain and subsequent dental treatment in Swedish adolescents. J Orofac Pain 2005; 19(2):144–50.

22. Aoyagi K, Goddard G, Karibe H, et al. Comparison of subjective symptoms of temporomandibular disorders in young patients by age and gender. Cranio 2012;30(2):114–20.

23. Greene CS. The etiology of temporomandibular disorders: implications for treatment. J Orofac Pain 2001;15(2):93–105.

24. Mohlin B, Axelsson S, Paulin G, et al. TMD in relation to malocclusion and orthodontic treatment. Angle Orthod 2007;77(3):542–8.

25. LeResche L. Epidemiology of temporomandibular disorders: implications for the investigation of etiologic factors. Crit Rev Oral Biol Med 1997;8:291–305.

26. Wadhwa S, Kapila S. TMJ disorders: future innovations in diagnostics and therapeutics. J Dent Educ 2008;72(8):930–47.

27. Nekora-Azak A, Evlioglu G, Ceyhan A, et al. Estrogen replacement therapy among postmenopausal women and its effects on signs and symptoms of temporomandibular disorders. Cranio 2008;26(3):211–5.

28. De Boever JA, Keersmaekers K. Trauma in patients with temporomandibular disorders: frequency and treatment outcome. J Oral Rehabil 1996;23(2):91–6.
29. Roda RP, Bagán JV, Díaz Fernández JM, et al. Review of temporomandibular joint pathology. Part I: classification, epidemiology and risk factors. Med Oral Patol Oral Cir Bucal 2007;12:E292–8.
30. Twilt M, Schulten AJ, Nicolaas P, et al. Concise report: facioskeletal changes in children with juvenile idiopathic arthritis. Ann Rheum Dis 2006;65:823–5.
31. Howard JA, Lovrovich AT. Wind instruments: their interplay with orofacial structures. Med Probl Perform Art 1989;4:59–72.
32. Kovero O, Könönen M. Signs and symptoms of temporomandibular disorders and radiologically observed abnormalities in the condyles of the temporomandibular joints of professional violin and viola players. Acta Odontol Scand 1995; 53(2):81–4.
33. Kovero O, Könönen M. Signs and symptoms of temporomandibular disorders in adolescent violin players. Acta Odontol Scand 1996;54(4):271–4.
34. Al-Ani Z, Gray R. TMD current concepts: an update. Dent Update 2007;34: 278–88.
35. Rugh JD, Woods BJ, Dahlström L. Temporomandibular disorders: assessment of psychological factors. Adv Dent Res 1993;7(2):127–36.
36. Carra MC, Huynh N, Morton P, et al. Prevalence and risk factors of sleep bruxism and wake-time tooth clenching in a 7- to 17-yr-old population. Eur J Oral Sci 2011; 119(5):386–94.
37. Thilander B, Rubio G, Pena L, et al. Prevalence of temporomandibular dysfunction and its association with malocclusion in children and adolescents: an epidemiologic study related to specified stages of dental development. Angle Orthod 2002;72(2):146–54.
38. Pullinger AG, Seligman DA. Quantification and validation of predictive values of occlusal variables in temporomandibular disorders using a multifactorial analysis. J Prosthet Dent 2000;83(1):66–75.
39. Türp JC, Schindler H. The dental occlusion as a suspected cause for TMDs: epidemiological and etiological consideration. J Oral Rehabil 2012;39(7):502–12.
40. Hirsch C, John MT, Stang A. Association between generalized joint hypermobility and signs and diagnoses of temporomandibular disorders. Eur J Oral Sci 2008; 116(6):525–30.
41. Huddleston Slater JJ, Lobbezoo F, Onland-Moret NC, et al. Anterior disc displacement with reduction and symptomatic hypermobility in the human temporomandibular joint: prevalence rates and risk factors in children and teenagers. J Orofac Pain 2007;21(1):55–62.
42. Akhter R, Hassan NM, Ohkubo R, et al. The relationship between jaw injury, third molar removal, and orthodontic treatment and TMD symptoms in university students in Japan. J Orofac Pain 2008;22(1):50–6.
43. Imahara SD, Hopper RA, Wang J, et al. Patterns and outcomes of pediatric facial fractures in the United States: a survey of the National Trauma Data Bank. J Am Coll Surg 2008;207(5):710–6.
44. Abou-Atme YS, Chedid N, Melis M, et al. Clinical measurement of normal maximum mouth opening in children. Cranio 2008;26(3):191–6.
45. Karlo CA, Stolzmann P, Habernig S, et al. Size, shape and age-related changes of the mandibular condyle during childhood. Eur Radiol 2010;20(10):2512–7.
46. Nebbe B, Major PW, Prasad N. Female adolescent facial pattern associated with TMJ disk displacement and reduction in disk length: part I. Am J Orthod Dentofacial Orthop 1999;116(2):168–76.

47. Dibbets JM, Carlson DS. Implications of temporomandibular disorders for facial growth and orthodontic treatment. Semin Orthod 1995;1(4):258–72.
48. Lei J, Liu MQ, Yap AU, et al. Condylar subchondral formation of cortical bone in adolescents and young adults. Br J Oral Maxillofac Surg 2012. http://dx.doi.org/10.1016/j.bjoms.2012.02.006.
49. Parker MW. A dynamic model of etiology in temporomandibular disorders. J Am Dent Assoc 1990;120:283–90.
50. Clark GT. Etiologic theory and the prevention of temporomandibular disorders. Adv Dent Res 1991;5:60–6.
51. Kleinrok M, Mielnik-Hus J, Zysko-Wozniak D, et al. Investigations on prevalence and treatment of fingernail biting. Cranio 1990;8:47–50.
52. Ito T, Gibbs CH, Bonnet RM, et al. Loading on the temporomandibular joints with five occlusal conditions. J Prosthet Dent 1986;56:478–84.
53. Ringold S, Cron RQ. The temporomandibular joint in juvenile idiopathic arthritis: frequently used and frequently arthritic. Pediatr Rheumatol Online J 2009;7:11.
54. Pearson MH, Rönning O. Lesions of the mandibular condyle in juvenile chronic arthritis. Br J Orthod 1996;23(1):49–56.
55. Weideman CL, Bush DL, Yan-Go FL, et al. The incidence of parasomnias in child bruxers versus nonbruxers. Pediatr Dent 1996;18(7):456–60.
56. Clark GT, Dionne RA. Orofacial pain: a guide to medications and management. Oxford (England): Wiley-Blackwell; 2012. p. 129–44.
57. Monroy PG, da Fonseca MA. The use of botulinum toxin-A in the treatment of severe bruxism in a patient with autism: a case report. Spec Care Dentist 2006;26(1):37–9.
58. Herpertz-Dahlmann B. Adolescent eating disorders: definitions, symptomatology, epidemiology and comorbidity. Child Adolesc Psychiatr Clin North Am 2009; 18(1):31–47.
59. Riad M, Barton JR, Wilson JA, et al. Parotid salivary secretory pattern in bulimia nervosa. Acta Otolaryngol 1991;111(2):392–5.
60. Robinson P, Grossi L. Gag reflex in bulimia nervosa. Lancet 1986;26(2):221–3.
61. Stegenga B. Nomenclature and classification of temporomandibular joint disorders. J Oral Rehabil 2010;37:760–5.
62. Dibbets JM, Dijkman GE. The postnatal development of the temporal part of the human temporomandibular joint. a quantitative study on skulls. Ann Anat 1997; 179(6):569–72.
63. Katsavrias EG. Changes in articular eminence inclination during the craniofacial growth period. Angle Orthod 2002;72(3):258–64.
64. Undt G, Kermer C, Piehslinger E, et al. Treatment of recurrent mandibular dislocation, part 1: Leclerc blocking procedure. Int J Oral Maxillofac Surg 1997;26(2):92–7.
65. Nitzan DW. Temporomandibular joint "open lock" versus condylar dislocation: signs and symptoms, imaging, treatment, and pathogenesis. J Oral Maxillofac Surg 2002;60(5):506–13.
66. Goddard G. Controversies in TMD. J Calif Dent Assoc 1998;11:827–32.
67. Von Korff MR, Howard JA, Truelove EL, et al. Temporomandibular disorders: variations in clinical practice. Med Care 1988;26:307–14.
68. Clark GT. A critical evaluation of orthopedic interocclusal appliance therapy, part 1: theory, design, and overall effectiveness. J Am Dent Assoc 1984;108:359–64.
69. Dao TT, Lavigne GJ. Oral splints: the crutches for temporomandibular disorders and bruxism? Crit Rev Oral Biol Med 1998;9(3):345–61.
70. Wurgaft R, Wong RK. Temporomandibular joint remodeling for the treatment of temporomandibular joint disorders: a clinical case study. Open Rehabil J 2009; 2:48–54.

71. Ettlin DA, Mang H, Colombo V, et al. Stereometric assessment of TMJ space variation by occlusal splints. J Dent Res 2008;87(9):877–81.
72. Stapelmann H, Türp JC. The NTI-tss device for the therapy of bruxism, temporomandibular disorders, and headache – where do we stand? A qualitative systematic review of the literature. BMC Oral Health 2008;8:22.
73. Kaban LB, Bouchard C, Troulis MJ. A protocol for management of temporomandibular joint ankylosis in children. J Oral Maxillofac Surg 2009;67(9):1966–78.
74. Gynther GQ, Holmlund AB. Efficacy of arthroscopic lysis and lavage in patients with temporomandibular joint symptoms associated with generalized osteoarthritis or rheumatoid arthritis. J Oral Maxillofac Surg 1998;56(2):147–51.
75. Roychoudhury A, Parkash H, Trikha A. Functional restoration by gap arthroplasty in temporomandibular joint ankylosis: a report of 50 cases. Oral Surg Oral Med Oral Pathol Oral Radiol Endod 1999;87(2):166–9.
76. Chrcanovic BR. Open versus closed reduction: mandibular condylar fractures in children. Oral Maxillofac Surg 2012;16(3):245–55.
77. Clinical Affairs Committee -Temporomandibular Joint Problems in Children Subcommittee. Guideline on acquired temporomandibular disorders in infants, children, and adolescents. Chicago (IL): American Academy of Pediatric Dentistry; 2010. Reference Manual 33(6):11/12.

The Continuum of Behavior Guidance

Travis Nelson, DDS, MSD, MPH

KEYWORDS

- Behavior guidance • Behavior management • Sedation • General anesthesia
- Patient-centered care

KEY POINTS

- Behavior guidance is a continuum of skills spanning from basic to advanced techniques. Providing care to children requires understanding of the full continuum.
- Patient assessment includes anticipation of parental expectations, child temperament, and technical procedures. It dictates the appropriate behavior guidance technique for each child.
- Basic behavior guidance encompasses communicative behavior guidance, audiovisual distraction, nitrous oxide/oxygen inhalation, and delayed or alternative restorative treatment.
- Advanced behavior guidance encompasses protective stabilization, sedation, and general anesthesia. Its use should be restricted to those who have advanced training.
- By implementing the appropriate behavior guidance strategy, a healing relationship is maintained and the child is equipped to receive dental treatment throughout their lifetime.

INTRODUCTION

Most treatments provided within the comprehensive dental care of children are relatively simple, yet many practitioners find that *delivering* high-quality care to young children is challenging, which is not because of the technical procedures that must be rendered, but because they are performed on a child. The provision of dental care to children presents unique challenges and opportunities. To effectively treat children, providers must be prepared to address child behavior and leverage appropriate behavior guidance techniques.

Behavior guidance eases fear and anxiety and promotes an understanding of the need for good oral health.[1] This two-way *therapeutic relationship* is fundamental to the strategies presented within this article. These strategies, known as the discipline of behavior guidance, are presented here as a continuum. Thoughtful and individualized selection of

---

Department of Pediatric Dentistry, University of Washington, 6222 Northeast 74th Street, Seattle, WA 98115, USA
E-mail address: tmnelson@uw.edu

Dent Clin N Am 57 (2013) 129–143
http://dx.doi.org/10.1016/j.cden.2012.09.006   **dental.theclinics.com**

the appropriate approach within this continuum determines the successful practice of pediatric dentistry.

AN OVERVIEW OF BEHAVIOR GUIDANCE

The American Academy of Pediatric Dentistry (AAPD) defines behavior guidance as:

> *"A continuum of interaction involving the dentist and dental team, the patient, and the parent directed toward communication and education."[1]*

The individual techniques in behavior guidance are categorized as *basic behavior guidance* and *advanced behavior guidance* (**Table 1**). This article does not discuss each element of behavior guidance in detail, but enables the reader to visualize each technique within the conceptual framework of a continuum (**Fig. 1**).

THE CONTINUUM OF BEHAVIOR GUIDANCE: PRINCIPLES OF PRACTICE

With time, each practitioner develops his or her own unique style of behavior guidance. This skill set is developed through perspective gained in training and clinical experience. A unique practice style is what distinguishes the provider as an individual and allows them to practice from a place of *conviction* and *authenticity*. Although each style of behavior guidance may vary, there are certain fundamental principles of practice that should not. For example,

- A positive, healing, *therapeutic relationship*[2] is maintained between the child, the parent, and the dentist. This healing relationship is predicated on trust, effective communication, empathy for the patient, and provider reliability.
- There is one diagnosis for a given condition, yet there are typically multiple acceptable treatment options. Child behavior may require variation in the *treatment provided.*
- Child behavior may dictate variation in the *methods used to deliver care.*
- Treatment that is not definitive may be performed to effectively treat the disease while preserving the therapeutic relationship.

These principles are the basis of patient-centered care. This approach requires that the practitioner address not only the disease but also the patient's experience of the illness.[3] In pediatric dentistry, this means that special precautions are taken to ensure that the diseased teeth are not just treated but cared for in a manner that is considerate of each child's individual needs-child centered care. In 1895, McElroy[4]

Table 1
Behavior guidance techniques

Behavior Guidance	
Basic	**Advanced**
Communication and Communicative Guidance	Protective stabilization
○ Tell-Show-Do	Sedation
○ Voice control	General anesthesia
○ Nonverbal communication	
○ Positive reinforcement	
○ Distraction	
○ Parental presence/absence	
Audiovisual distraction	
Nitrous oxide/oxygen inhalation	

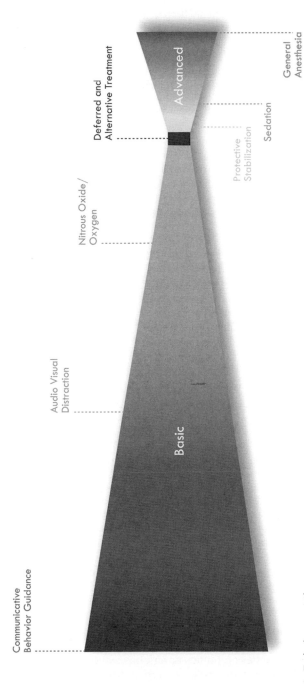

Fig. 1. Technique continuum.

recognized that "although the operative dentistry may be perfect, the appointment is a failure if the child departs in tears." If the tooth is saved but the patient's developing psyche is damaged in the process, child centered care was not provided.

The AAPD states that behavior guidance "is not an application of individual techniques created to deal with children, but rather a comprehensive, continuous method meant to develop and nurture the relationship between patient and doctor, which ultimately builds trust and allays fear and anxiety."[1] The aim should be not only to eliminate the immediate dental problem but also to equip the patient with the coping skills necessary to maintain optimal oral health throughout their lifetime.

PATIENT ASSESSMENT

To effectively provide pediatric dental care, a behavior guidance approach that is appropriate to each child is selected. The process of choosing the approach is as much an art as it is a science.[1] A well-balanced practitioner should possess a diverse skill set that can accommodate the wide variety of children who present to them for care. Thus, perhaps the most important skill that the clinician must master is *anticipation*. For example, it is imperative that the clinician anticipate:

- *Parenting style and expectations for dental care*. Some parents may refuse advanced behavior guidance such as sedation and general anesthesia (GA) for their child, whereas others demand it.
- *Child temperament and coping ability*. Some young children are not capable of coping with dental care in the clinic setting, whereas others sit peacefully during the operative procedures.
- *Technical procedures necessary to complete care*. The provider should anticipate those teeth that will require pulp therapy so that the materials will be on hand and the child is not made to wait for an excessively long period for the procedure to be completed.

An understanding of each of these elements will enable the dentist to select the treatment and behavior guidance method most appropriate to the child. It will also enable he or she to predict the potential behavioral complications before they arise, making accommodations to ensure a successful outcome.

THE PRETREATMENT PATIENT ASSESSMENT
Age-Appropriate Behavior

Children become more capable of accepting dental procedures as they grow older. Young children develop rapidly, and within six months, the child may be capable of tolerating procedures that they could not cope with earlier. This rapid development is the basis for the concept of deferred treatment. A 5-year-old child is often much more capable of receiving dental treatment than they were at age 3.5 or 4 years. However, if the treatment cannot be withheld without complications sedation or GA may be required (**Table 2**).

Medical History

Critical review of the medical history will enable the practitioner not only to avoid treatments which could be unsafe for the patient but also will provide them with information on the child's behavior. Particular emphasis should be placed on the psychological aspect of the history. Patients with autism, attention-deficit/hyperactivity disorder, or developmental delay present unique behavioral challenges. Items such as school performance, the ability to socialize, and the ability to tolerate haircuts

Table 2
Age-related psychosocial traits and skills for 2- to 5-year-old children

Age	Traits
Two	Likes to see and touch
	Very attached to parent
	Limited vocabulary with early sentence formation
Three	Less egocentric; likes to please
	Active imagination; likes stories
	Remains closely attached to parent
Four	Tries to impose powers
	Reaches out-expansive period
	Knows "thank you" and "please"
Five	Undergoes a period of consolidation, is deliberate
	Relinquishes comfort objects, such as a blanket or thumb

Adapted from McDonald RE, Avery DR, Dean JA. Dentistry for the child and adolescent. 8th edition. St. Louis (MO): Mosby; 2004; with permission.

and medical procedures can be predictive of a child's ability to cooperate in the dental office.[5]

Presentation of Oral Disease

The presentation of oral disease can be a critical factor in selecting the behavior guidance approach. Factors to consider include, among others, the urgency of the condition, location (ie, anterior vs posterior teeth), and the time to tooth exfoliation. Treatment may deferred on an asymptomatic primary anterior tooth of a 7-year-old because it is nearing exfoliation, but it may be advisable to treat the same lesion on a 3-year-old.

Temperament

Temperament is defined as the behavioral style of a child or the manner in which the child interacts with the environment. Temperament affects a child's behavior in a given situation. The clinician must match the temperament or behavioral style of the child with the environmental expectations and demands placed on them for a successful treatment.[6] This concept is called goodness of fit.[7] The implication is that those children who have an easy or adaptable temperament will often readily accept dental treatment. Likewise, those have more difficult temperament may have more difficulty tolerating dental treatment. Thus, the environmental expectations placed on them should be adjusted to fit their circumstances (ie, a different behavior guidance approach may be necessary for these children).[8] The more experience the clinician has working with children, the more capable he or she will become at evaluating child temperament. As the dentist's skill at evaluating child temperament improves, so does his or her ability to predict how well an individual child will cope with dental treatment. A brief evaluation should include:

- Child temperament (negative emotionality, activity, shyness, and impulsivity)[9,10]
- Behavioral problems (externalizing and internalizing)
- Attention or concentration problems[9]
- Verbal and behavioral interaction with the dentist
- Level of cooperation
- Level of attachment to parent[8,11]

Parent/Caregiver Preferences

Although the focus in pediatric dentistry is the child, the practitioner must also address the caregiver when providing treatment. Caregiver factors to consider include:

- His/her own anxiety regarding dental care and/or the child's appointment. Anxious parents may inadvertently transmit their emotions to the child, making it more difficult to complete care.
- Opinion on behavior-guidance techniques. Some parents of children with special health care needs refuse advanced behavior guidance such as immobilization, whereas others request that it be used for care.
- Preference of restorative materials. It may not be possible to use materials such as stainless steel crowns if they are thought by parents to be unacceptable for cosmetic reasons.
- Willingness to delay treatment versus desire for immediate definitive care. If the parent does not believe that he/she can return for the multiple follow-up preventive visits that are required in deferred treatment, comprehensive treatment using advanced behavior guidance may be preferable.
- Attitude toward oral health. The parent who has a fatalistic view of oral health does not believe that they have control over the disease outcome. Thus, their child may not be a good candidate for delayed treatment.

BASIC BEHAVIOR GUIDANCE STRATEGIES
Communicative Behavior Guidance

Most children who present for dental care can be treated using basic behavior guidance. The most fundamental of the basic strategies is *communicative behavior guidance*. This domain encompasses tell-show-do, voice control, nonverbal communication, positive reinforcement, and distraction.[1] Tell-show-do is a technique formalized over 5 decades ago. It is the cornerstone of behavior management: a series of successive approximations. By explaining and demonstrating procedures before doing them, the dentist gains the child's confidence.[12] Voice control is a communicative technique that focuses on the *delivery* of the message the child receives. It is defined "modulation in voice volume, tone, or pace to influence and direct a patient's behavior."[1] The modulation need not be in the direction of increased volume or a stern tone. In many cases lowering volume to a whisper is an effective way to gain the patient's attention and extinguish negative behavior. Positive reinforcement is the practice of shaping a patient's behavior through appropriately timed feedback and is used to reinforce helpful behaviors. Tangible reinforcements, such as prizes that a child receives at the completion of the dental visit, may also reinforce positive behavior and leave the child with a pleasant reminder of the dental appointment.

In appropriately applying communicative behavior guidance, it is imperative that the dentist interacts with the child at their developmental level.[14] The delivery of the message plays a critical role in each of the communicative behavior guidance strategies. More than 50% of communication is expressed nonverbally in movement, gesture, and timing.[15] Thus, the dentist's self-confidence, posture, and poise are as critical as the words he/she speaks. This effect has been described elsewhere as *calm-assertive energy*.[16] Often children misbehave because they are nervous or uncertain about being in the dental office. By adopting a calm-assertive approach, the dentist assures the child and maximizes the nonverbal aspects of communicative behavior guidance.

Audiovisual Distraction

Pain may be a cause for negative behavior in the dental chair.[17] Therefore, the clinician may attempt to distract the patient to decrease the discomfort they experience during the procedure. A growing body of evidence shows that audiovisual (AV) distraction (eg, movies, music, and video games) can be very effective in decreasing pain experience for medical procedures.[18–22] AV distraction has also been cited as a technological adjunct to traditional distraction techniques in the dental office.[23,24] Specific advantages of AV distraction are:

- The patient can choose their preferred distraction (movie/game)
- Concentration on the screen image distracts from the view of dental treatment
- Sound of the program may decrease or eliminate dental handpiece noise[24]

Despite its effectiveness in improving child behavior, AV distraction can also become problematic if the child is so immersed in the program that they cease to interact with the dentist. To minimize problems, the dentist must pay attention to appropriate program volume, continue to maintain communication with the child throughout the procedure, and reserve the right to remove the AV distraction should the child cease to follow instructions. AV distraction should be used in the same way as parental presence in the operatory; that is, if the child is cooperating and behaving appropriately the AV distraction is kept in place. If the child's behavior begins to deteriorate, the dentist should tell her that to continue viewing the monitor, she needs to be cooperative (eg, be quiet, open her mouth, and be still). This regulation sets appropriate boundaries and extinguishes inappropriate behavior.

Parental Presence/Absence

Historically in Pediatric Dentistry, children were commonly separated from their parents in the waiting area. As society has changed and as dentists have begun seeing younger and younger children, the number of parents who accompany children in the treatment area has also increased.[25] For some children separation from their parent may be emotionally challenging because they perceive their parent to be a source of comfort and protection.[26] This is the basis for the technique of parental presence/absence. As with all behavior guidance techniques, both the parent and practitioner must agree on this technique *before* it is put into practice. When used, the parent agrees to leave the treatment area if requested by the practitioner. The dentist offers the child that the parent can remain in the operatory as long as they exhibit good behavior. If the child displays negative behavior, the parent is asked to leave. This technique has proven to be an effective way to extinguish negative behaviors for some children.[27,28]

Nitrous Oxide/Oxygen Inhalation

Although it falls within the pharmacologic domain, nitrous oxide/oxygen inhalation (N_2O/O_2) is still considered basic behavior guidance. Nitrous oxide is an excellent and safe anxiolytic with analgesic properties, which provides the patient a pleasurable sensation of relaxation with possible symptoms of body warmth, tingling of the hands and feet, circumoral numbness, auditory effects, and euphoria. At levels of 40% N_2O it is suggested that it may produce good hard and soft tissue analgesia.[29,30] Although it is not typically a substitute for effective local anesthesia, when the provider anticipates that injection of local anesthetic may be the primary behavioral trigger, N_2O/O_2 can be effectively used in lieu of local anesthetic. One technique is to increase the relative percentage of nitrous oxide administered during components of the procedure, which could be more uncomfortable or which the child may have difficulty with, such as local anesthetic administration. In addition, for many patients N_2O/O_2 decreases the gag reflex.[31] Thus, although N_2O/O_2 does not replace other behavior guidance techniques, it may be a helpful adjunct for decreasing discomfort and anxiety.

Alternative Restorative Treatments

When working with children, barriers to treatment must be anticipated, and the approach should also be flexible. In some circumstances, given the age, extent of disease, parental preference, time to tooth exfoliation, or clinician's preference, conventional restorative treatment may not be possible or desirable. Alternative approaches may be considered in such circumstances. Alternative restorative treatments are not a specific behavior guidance technique; however, their use does fall within behavior guidance. In the continuum addressed here, alternative restorative treatments are positioned along with deferred treatment, immediately before the advanced behavior guidance techniques.

The interim therapeutic restoration (ITR) is a treatment that has been used in contemporary clinical practice because of such constraints. According to the AAPD,

> "ITR may be used to restore and prevent further decalcification in young patients, uncooperative patients, or patients with special health care needs, or when traditional cavity preparation and/or placement of traditional dental restorations are not feasible or need to be postponed."[32]

As stated previously, deferring treatment for even 6 months may in some cases allow a child to mature to the point where he/she is capable of receiving care. Furthermore, some ITR restorations may function adequately until natural exfoliation, never requiring re-treatment with traditional restorative techniques.

ITR is most typically done with fluoride-containing glass ionomer materials. Local anesthetic is often not used, and minimal tooth structure is removed. Decay often remains after tooth preparation. ITR has its greatest success when applied to single surface or small 2 surface restorations.[32] A meta-analysis showed survival rates for single-surface ITR-type restorations in primary teeth to be 95% at 2 years. Multi-surface restorations had 62% survival at 2 years, and sealants placed using the technique showed 1% new lesion incidence in the first 3 years.[33] ITR should be used with informed consent in combination with a caries preventive program, which should include dietary and oral hygiene counseling, increased frequency of dental recall, monitoring of adequate fluoride exposure, and application of antimicrobial agents (eg, povidone iodine, xylitol, and chlorhexidine).

A novel alternative restorative approach called the Hall Technique has been discussed recently in the dental literature. It uses preformed stainless steel crowns cemented with glass ionomer cement onto carious primary teeth-without local anesthesia, tooth preparation, or decay removal.[34] A well-designed randomized clinical trial shows that when used by general dentists in the United Kingdom, this technique produced outcomes superior to those of the conventional restorations placed. Parent, patient, and dentist satisfaction was also reported to be higher with this minimally invasive approach.[35]

Within weeks after placement, the restorations equilibrate and occlusion is acceptable to the child. In a randomized trial, placement of 118 Hall crowns (89%) was rated as causing no apparent discomfort to the child. Seventy seven percent of children, 83% of caregivers, and 81% of dentists surveyed expressed a preference for the technique over the conventional restorative treatment.[35] At 60 months, 92% of the restorations showed successful survival.[36]

The Hall Technique is a relatively new restorative concept, and currently there is only a small body of research supporting its use. Therefore, more well-designed studies are needed to reach a conclusion regarding its effectiveness. Although it is uncertain whether this technique produces results similar to those of stainless steel crowns placed in the conventional fashion, the 2- and 5-year randomized clinical trial findings do suggest that it may become an attractive alternative to traditional techniques, particularly with children for whom the delivery of treatment under local anesthesia is not possible or desirable.

ADVANCED BEHAVIOR GUIDANCE STRATEGIES

Although most children can be treated using basic behavior guidance, those children who are young, have extensive dental needs, have a difficult temperament, have intellectual disability, or who have had negative experiences in the past may require advanced behavior management.[1] This strategy includes protective stabilization, sedation, and GA. The advanced behavior guidance techniques commonly are used and taught in advanced pediatric dental training programs. Safe and effective implementation of these techniques requires knowledge and experience that is generally beyond the core knowledge that students receive during predoctoral dental education. Dentists considering the use of these advanced behavior guidance techniques should seek additional training through a residency program, a graduate program, and/or an extensive continuing education course that involves both didactic and experiential mentored training.[1]

Protective Stabilization

Protective stabilization is defined as "the restriction of a patient's freedom of movement, with or without the patient's permission, to decrease risk of injury while allowing safe completion of treatment."[1] This technique may be used judiciously to protect the patient, practitioner, staff, or parent during dental care. Use of protective stabilization is controversial, and all other treatment alternatives should be explored before using this technique. For some children with disabilities and for limited treatment (such as in an emergency), protective stabilization may be a helpful adjunct to other behavior guidance methods (**Table 3**).

Table 3 Indications and contraindications for the use of protective stabilization	
Protective Stabilization	
Indications	**Contraindications**
Patients who need immediate diagnosis or limited treatment and cannot cooperate because of age or intellectual disability	Cooperative nonsedated patients
Procedure cannot safely be accomplished without use of immobilization	Patients who cannot be immobilized because of medical or physical conditions, particularly those at risk for bone fracture, or organ/tissue damage (eg, Osteogenesis Imperfecta, epidermolysis bullosa)
Sedated patients who require stabilization to limit untoward movement	Patients who have experienced previous physical or psychological trauma from previous protective stabilization
	Nonsedated patients with nonemergent treatment requiring lengthy appointments

The cooperation of children for invasive dental treatment is surprising, given that it can be uncomfortable. Still, most children are capable of coping with dental treatment and actually look forward to visiting the dentist. Yet, for every child there may come a point when he or she is no longer capable of cooperating. For some children, that may be the first operative dental visit. For others, it may come after many visits. The practitioner must do their best to *anticipate* the child's ability to cope with treatment and make accommodations to match the delivery of treatment with a behavior management technique that will allow that child to receive dental care.

Learning to cope with dental treatment is an important life skill. Thus, there is great value in children learning to receive treatment in the dental office. There is little value, however, in subjecting a young child with limited coping skills to appointment after appointment of difficult operative procedures. Learning the skills necessary to receive dental examination, prophylaxis, radiographs, and simple operative treatment is beneficial for the child's long-term health. Learning the skills necessary to receive the procedures that full mouth rehabilitation requires is not something that many young children are capable of from a developmental standpoint. Attempting to provide this type of care to young children using only basic behavior management will almost certainly push the child past the point where they are capable of coping, traumatizing the child, breaking the therapeutic relationship, and causing the dentist to fail in providing child-centered care. If a child is so frightened of dentistry that good behavior is impossible, it is the dentist's obligation to avoid increasing the child's anxieties. This may mean using alternative restorative treatments to postpone nonurgent dental work or using sedation or GA.[13]

Sedation

Sedation can be very useful in preventing or reducing behavioral issues that arise as a result of discomfort and anxiety related to the dental appointment. Additionally some sedative agents can cause amnesia, which is desirable if a difficult procedure or a long appointment is anticipated.[10] As mentioned before, behavior guidance is a continuum. Similarly, the pharmacologic behavioral guidance techniques of sedation and GA form a continuum. It is important to recognize that some patients only require very mild levels of sedation, whereas others will not cooperate without deep sedation or GA (**Box 1**).

Box 1
Indications for sedation

Fearful, anxious patients for whom basic behavior guidance has not been successful and those children with a past history of uncooperative behavior

Patients who cannot cooperate because of a lack of psychological or emotional maturity and/or mental, physical, or medical disability

Patients for whom the use of sedation may protect the developing psyche and/or reduce medical risk

Young patents whom are minimally cooperative, or pre-cooperative

Those children with extensive treatment needs for whom repeated treatment may cause psychological or emotional trauma

Children who travel extensive distance to receive care

Data from American Academy of Pediatric Dentistry Clinical Affairs Committee. Guideline on behavior guidance for the pediatric dental patient; 2011. p. 161–73.

The goal of sedation as practiced within the dental office should not be to pharmacologically immobilize the child, but rather to alleviate anxiety associated with the procedure, allowing the child's natural coping mechanisms to function. Thus, the intended level of sedation is mild-to-moderate. In the dental office, particularly with pediatric patients, this level of sedation is most typically achieved by oral administration. Although extremely common, the oral route of administration is inherently unpredictable, both in mental and physiologic effects. Published data show success of oral sedation ranging from 30% to 70%.[37] A practitioner who provides sedation must *anticipate* the intended level of sedation that a delivered dose will provide and take corrective action should the patient become more deeply sedated.

As with all other behavior guidance techniques, mastery of this domain hinges on *anticipation*. The chances of sedation success can be increased by carefully selecting the patients who receive it. For example, a very stubborn or uncooperative child may not be a good candidate for oral sedation. Safe administration of a sedative dose to allow the child to receive dental treatment is not possible because it would likely be in excess of the maximum recommended dosage, which could put the patient dangerously close to deep sedation or GA. Similarly, the child must also allow the administration of the drug. Those children who do not predictably take medications seldom prove to be good candidates for in-office sedation. As with other areas of dentistry, sedation inherently has both risks and benefits. Careful case selection prevents subjecting children who are poor sedation candidates to increased risk of medical complications from sedation.

In the preoperative assessment for sedation, it is critical to perform a thorough physical evaluation and to adequately assess the child's behavior and temperament. A pretreatment assessment of temperament and behavior is perhaps even more critical for children who are potential sedation candidates than for other pediatric patients. Child temperament subscales of approachability and adaptability are important predictive variables for children's behaviors.[6,8,38,39] Factors such as the child's response to change, new environments, an unknown adult, and shyness seem to be pivotal in predicting a child's behavior during the sedation visit.[10,11,40] A negative mood and general emotional/behavioral problems are also predictive of unsuccessful sedation outcomes.[9,38,41] Children who have more negative emotionality (ie, fear, anger) have a tendency to become more easily and intensely upset, which may reduce the amnestic effect of some medications.[10] Thus, it is possible to anticipate that children with some temperament types may be more wary and less likely to accept the influence of sedative medications. By carefully evaluating the whole child, the practitioner can increase the chances for successful sedation while providing safe and effective care.

GA

GA is defined as a controlled state of unconsciousness accompanied by a loss of protective reflexes, including the ability to maintain an airway independently and respond purposefully to physical stimulation and verbal commands (**Table 4**).[1] GA represents the far end of the behavior guidance continuum. Except in rare circumstances, it is possible to accomplish dental care for any child under GA. GA does not require cooperation from the child, as other modalities do, and thus may be desirable for very young children with extensive disease, those who are extremely uncooperative, fearful, anxious, and those with impaired cognitive abilities.

Despite the effectiveness of GA, it may not be the most desirable behavior guidance option. Factors to consider in case selection for GA include the amount of treatment required, urgency, parent preference, provider training, cost, and availability of GA

Table 4
Indications and contraindications for GA

General Anesthesia	
Indications	Contraindications
Patients who cannot cooperate because of a lack of psychological or emotional maturity and/or mental, physical, or medical disability	A healthy, cooperative patient with minimal dental needs
Patients for whom local anesthesia is ineffective because of acute infection, anatomic variations, or allergy	Predisposing medical conditions, which would make general anesthesia inadvisable
The extremely uncooperative, fearful, anxious, or uncommunicative child or adolescent	
Patients requiring significant surgical procedures	
Patients for whom the use of general anesthesia may protect the developing psyche and/or reduce medical risk	
Patients requiring immediate, comprehensive oral/dental care	

services.[42,43] For example, a young child with minimal nonurgent treatment needs may not be a good candidate for GA. The practitioner must determine which items of treatment are mandatory and which are optional. An abscessed tooth requires urgent care; however, it may be possible to postpone treatment of small caries lesions. In cases such as these, using alternative restorative techniques and addressing the disease process with antimicrobials and fluoride may be an attractive choice. On the continuum of behavior guidance, GA is the final treatment option; one that should be exercised with due consideration. In some cases it is the only viable alternative; however, it may be possible to address the disease process by using basic behavior guidance techniques that reside further down on the continuum.

Cost must also be considered. GA services typically cost thousands of dollars per child, and care must be exercised in their use.[42] When these services are in excess of what a patient's family can afford, the dentist may be required to consider other options. GA cost for dental services has been examined in research, but because of multiple complicating factors, the actual cost efficacy in comparison with the other treatment methods is not fully clear. One study cited 47% lower cost using sedation instead of GA; however, it was not clear what the cost effect would be if multiple visits were required.[44] Another project suggested that if the number of visits needed is greater than 3, GA offers cost savings over sedation.[42] The cost of services seems to be highly variable and depends significantly on the location and venue in which they are provided.[45]

In caring for the child patient, the dentist must rely on the parent or caregiver to make decisions regarding treatment. Because of the risks and benefits associated with GA, it is imperative that the provider and the parent be in agreement regarding the treatment approach. Parents may have strong opinions regarding the use of GA services in a growing child or the risks associated with this type of treatment. Those opinions should be clearly determined when choosing a treatment approach.

GA services may not be possible in all locations. Some dentists may not have access to them, and not all may be trained or comfortable working with that skill set. In those cases, it will be necessary to refer to another provider who uses other behavior guidance approaches to accomplish care.[43]

SUMMARY

Behavior guidance is fundamental to the provision of quality dental care for pediatric patients. The skills contained within this discipline represent a continuum. Clinicians must have a thorough understanding of this continuum and should be prepared to use a wide array of behavior guidance techniques. In pediatrics, the therapeutic relationship between patient and provider is the basis for the concept of child-centered care. By effectively using techniques within the continuum of behavior guidance, it is possible to honor this relationship while addressing dental disease. The ultimate goal is to maintain the healing relationship and empower each child with the coping skills to receive dental treatment throughout their lifetime.

REFERENCES

1. American Academy of Pediatric Dentistry. Guideline on behavior guidance for the pediatric dental patient. 2011:161–73.
2. Nash DA. Engaging children's cooperation in the dental environment through effective communication. Pediatr Dent 2006;28(5):455–9.
3. Bedos C, Loignon C. Patient-centred approaches: new models for new challenges. J Can Dent Assoc 2011;77:b88.
4. McElroy CM. Dentistry for Children: Calif Dent Assoc Trans 1895:85.
5. Marshall J, Sheller B, Williams BJ, et al. Cooperation predictors for dental patients with autism. Pediatr Dent 2007;29:369–76.
6. Lochary ME, Wilson S, Griffen AL, et al. Temperament as a predictor of behavior for conscious sedation in dentistry. Pediatr Dent 1993;15(5):348–52.
7. Carey WB, Fox M, McDevitt SC. Temperament as a factor in early school adjustment. Pediatrics 1977;60(4 Pt 2):621–4.
8. Radis FG, Wilson S, Griffen AL, et al. Temperament as a predictor of behavior during initial dental examination in children. Pediatr Dent 1994;16(2):121–7.
9. Arnrup K, Broberg AG, Berggren U, et al. Lack of cooperation in pediatric dentistry–the role of child personality characteristics. Pediatr Dent 2002;24(2):119–28.
10. Jensen B, Stjernqvist K. Temperament and acceptance of dental treatment under sedation in preschool children. Acta Odontol Scand 2002;60(4):231–6.
11. Fraone G, Wilson S, Casamassimo PS, et al. The effect of orally administered midazolam on children of three age groups during restorative dental care. Pediatr Dent 1999;21(4):235–41.
12. Addelston H. Child patient training. Fortn Rev Chic Dent Soc 1959;7–9, 27–9.
13. Pinkham JR, Casamassimo PS, Fields HW, et al. Pediatric dentistry infancy through adolescence. 4th edition. St. Louis (MO): Elsevier Saunders; 2005. p. 395–413.
14. McDonald RE, Avery DR, Dean JA. Dentistry for the child and adolescent. 8th edition. St. Louis (MO): Mosby; 2004. p. 35–49.
15. Mehrabian AA. Communication without words. Psychol Today 1968.
16. Millan C, Peltier MJ. Cesar's way. New York: Three Rivers Press; 2006. p. 59–78.
17. Nutter DP. Good clinical pain practice for pediatric procedure pain: target considerations. J Calif Dent Assoc 2009;37(10):719–22.
18. Das DA, Grimmer KA, Sparnon AL, et al. The efficacy of playing a virtual reality game in modulating pain for children with acute burn injuries: a randomized controlled trial [ISRCTN87413556]. BMC Pediatr 2005;5(1):1.
19. Kipping B, Rodger S, Miller K, et al. Virtual reality for acute pain reduction in adolescents undergoing burn wound care: a prospective randomized controlled trial. Burns 2012;38(5):650–7.

20. Maani CV, Hoffman HG, Morrow M, et al. Virtual reality pain control during burn wound debridement of combat-related burn injuries using robot-like arm mounted VR goggles. J Trauma 2011;71(Suppl 1):S125–30.
21. Miller K, Rodger S, Bucolo S, et al. Multi-modal distraction. Using technology to combat pain in young children with burn injuries. Burns 2010;36(5):647–58.
22. Morris LD, Louw QA, Grimmer-Somers K. The effectiveness of virtual reality on reducing pain and anxiety in burn injury patients: a systematic review. Clin J Pain 2009;25(9):815–26.
23. Ram D, Shapira J, Holan G, et al. Audiovisual video eyeglass distraction during dental treatment in children. Quintessence Int 2010;41(8):673–9.
24. Prabhakar AR, Marwah N, Raju OS. A comparison between audio and audiovisual distraction techniques in managing anxious pediatric dental patients. J Indian Soc Pedod Prev Dent 2007;25(4):177–82.
25. Ramos ME, Kao JY, Houpt M. Attitudes of pediatric dentists toward parental presence during dental treatment of children. J N J Dent Assoc 2010;81(3):32–7.
26. Frankl S, Shiere F, Fogels H. Should the parent remain with the child in the dental operatory? J Dent Child 1962;150–63.
27. Kotsanos N, Arhakis A, Coolidge T. Parental presence versus absence in the dental operatory: a technique to manage the uncooperative child dental patient. Eur J Paediatr Dent 2005;6(3):144–8.
28. Kotsanos N, Coolidge T, Velonis D, et al. A form of 'parental presence/absence' (PPA) technique for the child patient with dental behaviour management problems. Eur Arch Paediatr Dent 2009;10:90–2.
29. Yagiela JA, Dowd FJ, Neidle EA. Pharmacology and therapeutics for dentistry. 5th edition. St. Louis (MO): Elsevier Mosby; 2004. p. 287–9, 773–5.
30. Yagiela J. The pediatric patient and nitrous oxide. Dimens Dent Hyg 2008; 20–2.
31. Kaufman E, Weinstein P, Sommers EE, et al. An experimental study of the control of the gag reflex with nitrous oxide. Anesth Prog 1988;35(4):155–7.
32. American Academy on Pediatric Dentistry Council on Clinical Affairs. Policy on interim therapeutic restorations (ITR). Pediatr Dent 2008;30(Suppl 7):38–9.
33. de Amorim RG, Leal SC, Frencken JE. Survival of atraumatic restorative treatment (ART) sealants and restorations: a meta-analysis. Clin Oral Investig 2012;16(2): 429–41.
34. Innes NP, Stirrups DR, Evans DJ, et al. A novel technique using preformed metal crowns for managing carious primary molars in general practice–a retrospective analysis. Br Dent J 2006;200:451–4 [discussion: 44].
35. Innes NP, Evans DJ, Stirrups DR. The Hall Technique; a randomized controlled clinical trial of a novel method of managing carious primary molars in general dental practice: acceptability of the technique and outcomes at 23 months. BMC Oral Health 2007;7:18.
36. Innes NP, Evans DJ, Stirrups DR. Sealing caries in primary molars: randomized control trial, 5-year results. J Dent Res 2011;90(12):1405–10.
37. Lourenco-Matharu L, Ashley PF, Furness S. Sedation of children undergoing dental treatment. Cochrane Database Syst Rev 2012;(3):CD003877.
38. Cohen LL, Francher A, MacLaren JE, et al. Correlates of pediatric behavior and distress during intramuscular injections for invasive dental procedures. J Clin Pediatr Dent 2006;31(1):44–7.
39. Voepel-Lewis T, Malviya S, Prochaska G, et al. Sedation failures in children undergoing MRI and CT: is temperament a factor? Paediatr Anaesth 2000;10(3): 319–23.

40. Quinonez R, Santos RG, Boyar R, et al. Temperament and trait anxiety as predictors of child behavior prior to general anesthesia for dental surgery. Pediatr Dent 1997;19(6):427–31.
41. Arnrup K, Berggren U, Broberg AG, et al. A short-term follow-up of treatment outcome in groups of uncooperative child dental patients. Eur J Paediatr Dent 2004;5(4):216–24.
42. Lee J, Vann W, Roberts M. A cost analysis of treating pediatric dental patients using general anesthesia versus conscious sedation. Pediatr Dent 2000;22: 27–32.
43. Boyle CA. Sedation or general anaesthesia for treating anxious children. Evid Based Dent 2009;10(3):69.
44. Jameson K, Averley PA, Shackley P, et al. A comparison of the 'cost per child treated' at a primary care-based sedation referral service, compared to a general anaesthetic in hospital. Br Dent J 2007;203(6):E13.
45. Ashley PF, Williams CE, Moles DR, et al. Sedation versus general anaesthesia for provision of dental treatment in under 18 year olds. Cochrane Database Syst Rev 2009;(1):CD006334.

The Role of Sedation in Contemporary Pediatric Dentistry

Travis Nelson, DDS, MSD, MPH*, Gary Nelson, DDS, MS

KEYWORDS

- Pediatric dentistry • Sedation • Behavior guidance • General anesthesia

KEY POINTS

- Appropriate use of procedural sedation requires thorough knowledge of its indications and contraindications, as well as alternative methods of treatment.
- Sedation and general anesthesia represent a continuum. Individual responses to medication may cause variation in sedation depth.
- Patient selection for procedural sedation includes evaluation of treatment needs, child behavior, medical history, and physical assessment.
- Vigilant monitoring is key to safe, successful care. The ability to recognize adverse events early and intervene to rescue a child is fundamental to patient safety.
- Effective office protocol enables the practitioner to provide safe and efficient care.

INTRODUCTION

Children frequently present to the dentist with treatment needs that require invasive procedures. Procedural sedation can offer an effective and humane way to facilitate delivery of dental care to the young, anxious child and those with extensive treatment needs. To safely provide dentistry using sedation, it is crucial that the provider have a thorough understanding of sedation indications (**Box 1**), contraindications (**Box 2**), patient assessment, pharmacology, monitoring, protocol, and the ability to rescue a patient from unintended levels of sedation.

Use of Sedation in Pediatric Dentistry

It is generally accepted that the majority of children can receive dental treatment through nonpharmacologic behavioral guidance; however, some children require alternative approaches. In graduate pediatric dentistry programs in the United States it is estimated that 1% to 20% of the children treated require sedation, with most

Department of Pediatric Dentistry, University of Washington, 6222 Northeast 74th Street, Seattle, WA 98115, USA
* Corresponding author.
E-mail address: tmnelson@uw.edu

Dent Clin N Am 57 (2013) 145–161
http://dx.doi.org/10.1016/j.cden.2012.09.007
0011-8532/13/$ – see front matter © 2013 Elsevier Inc. All rights reserved.

Box 1
Indications for sedation

Fearful, anxious patients for whom basic behavior guidance has not been successful and those children with a past history of uncooperative behavior

Patients who cannot cooperate due to a lack of psychological or emotional maturity and/or mental, physical, or medical disability

Patients for whom the use of sedation may protect the developing psyche and/or reduce medical risk

Young patients whom are minimally cooperative, or pre-cooperative

Those children with extensive treatment needs for whom repeated treatment may cause psychological or emotional trauma

Children who travel extensive distance to receive care

Data from American Academy of Pediatric Dentistry Clinical Affairs Committee. Guideline on behavior guidance for the pediatric dental patient; 2011. p. 161–73.

---

program directors reporting an increase in the number of sedations performed annually.[1] Practice surveys of pediatric dentists also indicate an overall increased use of sedation for pediatric dentistry, with an estimated 100,000 to 250,000 pediatric dental sedations performed each year.[2–4] Dentists also report that children now exhibit more challenging behaviors than in the past, increasing the need for sedation.[5,6] The increase in the use of procedural sedation by practitioners with varied educational and practice backgrounds has simultaneously driven public and governmental demand for regulation and education to improve patient safety.

Historical Perspective

In 1983, in response to sedation incident reports from dental settings, the American Academy of Pediatrics (AAP) first requested that the section on Anesthesiology and the Committee on Drugs work with the American Academy of Pediatric Dentistry (AAPD) to formulate guidelines for pediatric sedation. In 1992, the AAP guidelines were revised to reflect advances in technology, requiring pulse oximetry for all sedated

---

Box 2
Contraindications and barriers to sedation

Cooperative patients with minimal dental needs

Patients with predisposing medical and/or physical conditions that would make sedation inadvisable

Parental objection or choice of an alternative option for treatment

Financial barriers

Language or cultural barriers

Inadequate training to provide safe care using sedation

Data from American Academy of Pediatric Dentistry Clinical Affairs Committee. Guideline on behavior guidance for the pediatric dental patient; 2011. p. 161–73.

children for the first time.[7] Several revisions have since occurred. The guidelines established by the AAP/AAPD are now the standard of care accepted by the Joint Commission on Accreditation of Healthcare Organizations (JCAHO) and others.[7,8]

THE ROLE OF SEDATION
Factors to Consider in Pharmacologic Guidance

When considering a pharmacologic approach to behavior guidance, the following factors should be considered:

- Risks involved with pharmacologic guidance compared with routine communicative techniques
- Extent of the patient's dental needs
- Practitioner training and experience, including the ability to "rescue" a child when significantly compromised
- Monitoring
- Cost and third-party payers
- Venue issues (ie, office vs outpatient care facility, rural vs urban)
- Parental expectations
- Nature of the child's cognitive/emotional needs and personality[6]

Alternatives to Sedation

In sedation, as with any area of dentistry, no treatment is an option that should be presented to the parent or guardian. Deferred treatment is another strategy that may be considered. Deferring treatment may allow the child to mature and accept treatment. The child may also benefit from behavior modification or progressive desensitization. In such cases it is advisable to implement a caries management protocol. This protocol may include dietary and oral hygiene counseling, increased frequency of recall, monitoring of adequate fluoride exposure and professional fluoride application, as well as application of antimicrobial agents (eg, povidone iodine, xylitol, and chlorhexidine).[9-12] Interim therapeutic restorations (ITR) may also be used to slow decay progression.[13]

For children who are not good candidates for deferred treatment or behavior modification, general anesthesia (GA) is an effective option. However, in some situations it may not be the most desirable option despite its effectiveness. Factors to consider include the amount of treatment required, urgency, cost, parent preference, provider training, and the availability of GA services.[14,15]

Goals of Sedation

- Guard the patient's safety and welfare. This goal is foremost, and is best accomplished by minimizing complications.
- Minimize physical discomfort.
- Minimize negative psychological responses to treatment by providing analgesia and anxiolysis, and maximizing the potential for amnesia.
- Provide quality dental care in an efficient manner that respects the child and the caregiver's time.[16-18]

THE CONTINUUM OF SEDATION AND ANESTHESIA
Individual Variation in Response to Sedative Medications

In the original guidelines established by the AAP, procedural sedation was referred to as conscious sedation. Over time, this term has fallen out of favor, being considered an oxymoron. Indeed, it has been stated that there is no such thing as "just a little sedation." In response, the 2002 AAP guideline replaced this term with the more precise label sedation/analgesia.[8] It is now recognized that practitioners who provide this service must be prepared to manage an unconscious child, should the sedation level unintentionally deepen.[19] Current recommendations describe sedation and GA not as separate entities but as a continuum.[19] Environmental, genetic, and individual patient factors affect the absorption, distribution, metabolism, and excretion of a given drug. Physiologic and behavioral responses also vary. The interplay of these factors determines the profile of the drug plasma concentration over time, and its elicited physiologic effect.

Some children may be hyper- or hyporesponders to a drug administered at a level that is therapeutic for the majority of the population.[20] The patient is best served by an alert provider, aware of the possibility that individual variation may create an unexpected drug response. If an adverse event occurs, the practitioner must be capable of rescuing the patient from a depth of sedation at least one level greater than the intended level.[19,21] For instance, practitioners intending moderate sedation/analgesia must be able to manage patients who enter a state of deep sedation/analgesia (**Table 1**).[22,23]

PATIENT SELECTION
Treatment Needs

The risk of untoward effects outweighs the benefit of sedation for patients with minimal treatment needs. Patients with extensive treatment needs, those who need immediate medical treatment, and those for whom local anesthesia is not effective may also not be good candidates. Examples of cases for which alternatives to procedural sedation should be considered are:

- The young child with incipient caries lesions
  - Alternative: Implement caries management protocol and ITR restorations, and monitor lesions until cooperation improves
- The child who has not fasted and needs emergency dental treatment
  - Alternative: Offer nitrous oxide/oxygen anxiolysis and local anesthesia. Protective stabilization may also be considered in the appropriate circumstances.
- The child for whom effective local anesthesia is not possible (severe local infection, hematological instability, history of unsuccessful local anesthesia)
  - Alternative: GA after obtaining proper medical consultations

Behavioral Assessment

Although extremely common, the oral route of sedation produces results that are inherently unpredictable. Published data show success of oral sedation ranging from 30% to 70%.[24,25] By evaluating child behavior, it is possible to select cases with a high likelihood of success.

- *Cognitive development.* The ability to assess each child's developmental level is crucial to case selection. Sedation is a behavior guidance adjunct, typically requiring the practitioner to interact verbally with the child during treatment. A low level of verbal interaction and ability to cooperate may be anticipated from young children, whereas the school age or teenage patient may have a much greater level of understanding and interaction. Thus, for successful outcomes with younger children a more profound level of sedation may be required. The older child should interact as a "member of the team," understanding the critical importance of his willingness to cooperate once sedated.

Table 1
Definitions of sedation (effective 01/01/2001) adapted from the American Society of Anesthesiologists and Joint Commission on Accreditation of Healthcare Organizations

Minimal Sedation "Anxiolysis"	⇨ Moderate Sedation "Conscious Sedation"	⇨ Deep Sedation/Analgesia	⇨ General Anesthesia
Responds normally to verbal stimulation	Responds purposefully to verbal commands, alone or accompanied by light tactile stimulus	Patient cannot easily be aroused, but responds purposefully following repeated or painful stimulation	Drug-induced loss of consciousness during which patients are not arousable, even by painful stimulation
Cognitive function and coordination may be impaired	No interventions are required to maintain a patent airway, spontaneous ventilation is adequate	Ability to independently maintain ventilatory function may be impaired; may require assistance in maintaining a patent airway—spontaneous ventilation may be inadequate	Ability to independently maintain ventilatory function is often impaired; often require assistance in maintaining a patent airway
Ventilatory and cardiovascular functions unaffected	Cardiovascular function is usually maintained	Cardiovascular function is usually maintained	Cardiovascular function may be impaired
Typical of patients sedated with N_2O/O_2	Intended level for most dental oral sedation	Typical of patients who are "oversedated" in the dental office	

Data from The Joint Commission. Comprehensive accreditation manual for hospitals: The official handbook. Oakbrook Terrace, IL: Joint Commission Resources; 2011; and The Joint Commission. Revisions to anesthesia care standards. Comprehensive accreditation manual for ambulatory care. Oakbrook Terrace, IL: Joint Commission Resources 2012.

- *Child temperament and personality*. This aspect is perhaps the most critical in selecting successful cases. Factors such as the child's adaptability to change, new environments, an unknown adult, and shyness appear to be pivotal in predicting his behavior during the sedation visit.[26–31] A negative mood (ie, fear, anger) and general emotional/behavioral problems are predictive of unsuccessful sedation outcomes.[32–34] Children with negative mood also have a tendency to become more easily and intensely upset, which may reduce the amnestic effect of some medications.[26]
- In practice, patients who are anxious but generally cooperative for simple dental procedures (dental prophylaxis, intraoral radiographs, and so forth) often make very good sedation candidates. Children who accept oral medications well and those who are not "clingy" to parents also make good candidates. It has been demonstrated that parents do a reasonable job of predicting their own child's response to new challenges, and their opinion may prove helpful during the behavioral assessment.[35]

Medical History

Review of systems

- General: The type and severity of underlying medical problems, quantified with the American Society of Anesthesiologists (ASA) physical status classification (**Table 2**), must be assessed. Patients in ASA classes I and II are candidates for in-office sedation.[36]
- Age: Patients younger than 12 months (some suggest 24 months) may pose excessive risk for in-office sedation.[37,38]

Table 2
American Society of Anesthesiologists physical status classification

		Examples	Suitability for Sedation
I	Healthy patient	Unremarkable past medical history	Excellent
II	Patient with mild systemic disease, no functional limitation	Mild asthma, controlled seizure disorder, anemia	Generally good
III	Patient with severe systemic disease, definite functional limitation	Moderate to severe asthma, poorly controlled seizure disorder, pneumonia, moderate obesity	Intermediate to poor: contraindicated for in-office dental sedation
IV	Patient with severe systemic disease that is a constant threat to life	Severe bronchopulmonary dysplasia, sepsis, advanced degrees of pulmonary, cardiac, hepatic, renal, or endocrine insufficiency	Poor: benefits do not outweigh risks
V	Moribund patient who is not expected to survive without intervention	Septic shock, severe trauma	Extremely poor
VI	A declared brain-dead patient whose organs are being removed for donation		

Data from Refs.[36,38,43]

- Cardiovascular: Patients with known cardiovascular disease (eg, congenital cyanotic heart disease, heart failure, dysrhythmias) are not good candidates, as most drugs used for sedation and analgesia can cause vasodilation and hypotension.
- Respiratory: Pulmonary disease, especially upper respiratory infections, must be assessed by lung auscultation. Risk of respiratory complications including laryngospasm is significantly elevated in patients with active respiratory illness. Respiratory disorders (eg, asthma, bronchopulmonary dysplasia, and premature birth) are relative contraindications because these conditions may impair the patient's ability to maintain adequate oxygenation during the procedure.[39–42]
- Airway: Airway abnormalities (eg, tracheomalacia, congenital abnormalities, obese patients, children who snore, and those with craniofacial syndromes) are relative contraindications, as these conditions may predispose the patient to airway obstruction.
- Neurologic/developmental: Psychiatric diagnosis such as autism or attention-deficit/hyperactivity disorder can make sedation unpredictable. Neurologic conditions such as seizures require a consultation with the patient's physician, because medications used for sedation may alter the patient's neurologic status.
- Gastrointestinal: Abnormalities of the gastrointestinal system should be noted, as they may modify absorption and distribution of oral medications. Such conditions may be relative contraindications.
- Hepatic and renal: The presence of hepatic or renal abnormality may affect absorption and distribution of oral medications, and are relative contraindications.[43]
- Obesity: Obese patients may have underlying respiratory issues, obstructive sleep apnea, limited intravenous access (needed in the event of an emergency), and altered drug metabolism and distribution.
- Pregnancy status: Because most sedation medications are contraindicated during pregnancy, pregnancy status should be verified in women of childbearing age before administration of sedation medications.[44–46]
- Prior history of sedation or GA: A thorough history of the patient's experience with sedation and/or GA will determine if any adverse events have occurred in the past.[42]

Medications

All of the patient's prescription and nonprescription drugs and supplements should be accounted for, as they may affect medications used in sedation or may be affected by them.[47] Older patients should also be questioned regarding illicit drug use, as these substances may also cause potentially harmful side effects in combination with sedative agents.[48,49] Allergies and any history of adverse drug reactions should also be considered.

Physical Assessment

- Airway: Airway patency is a critical aspect of the presedation physical assessment. Relative percentage of tonsillar obstruction as evaluated by Brodsky classification is a good predictor of potential airway obstruction. Patients rated as III+ or greater may not be good sedation candidates (**Fig. 1**).
- Brodsky classification: Tonsillar obstruction[50,51]
  - 0, tonsils absent
  - I+, <25%
  - II+, 25%–50%
  - III+, 50%–75%
  - IV+, >75%

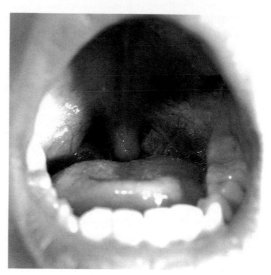

Fig. 1. Airway assessment.

- Respiratory system: Verify that respiratory rate is within normal parameters for the patient's age. Patients who are good candidates should have no history of recent respiratory illness and clear lung sounds on auscultation.
- Cardiovascular system: Assess by auscultation for structural abnormalities that could present as a murmur. The patient's heart rate, blood pressure, and blood oxygen saturation should also be verified as within normal limits.
- Weight: Record the patient's weight on the day of treatment. Some practitioners recommend subtracting 1 kg to account for clothing.
- General impression: Make a general assessment of the child. He should appear healthy, and without any unusual facial or physical characteristics. These observations may not otherwise be reflected in the physical examination, but could prove to be important.

ROUTES OF SEDATION

Although oral sedation is most common, several other options exist. Each route has unique advantages and disadvantages as well as federal and state oversight requirements (**Table 3**).

MONITORING

Administration of a sedative agent can decrease the patient's ability to maintain normal physiology and protective reflexes. Thus, the primary safeguard against adverse sedation events is vigilant patient monitoring and quick corrective action when indicated.

The Human Monitor

When moderate sedation is the intended end point, at least one person in addition to the practitioner must be present. His or her responsibility is to monitor physiologic parameters and to assist in any supportive or resuscitation measures if required. The monitor should have a minimum competency of basic life support training.[8] The clinician's eyes

Table 3
Sedation routes

Route	Training/Permit Requirements	Onset	Titration	Advanced Training/Permit Required
Inhalation	In office this is most typically used for nitrous oxide/oxygen only	Rapid onset and recovery	Yes	No
Intravenous (IV)	Technically demanding to administer	Rapid onset	Yes	Yes
Intramuscular (IM)	Less technically demanding to administer than IV	Variable onset dependent on local factors	No	Yes
Subcutaneous/ submucosal	Similar to skill set required for IM injection	Variable onset	No	Yes
Intranasal	Administration is minimally technically demanding	Typically more rapid than oral route, without first-pass metabolism	No	May be required
Oral	Administration is not technically demanding	Variable onset (10–90 min)	No May not redose, even if child spits out medication	May not be required for single agent

and ears must also function as a primary sedation monitor. Head position, breath sounds, chest movement, and patient color should be evaluated continuously throughout the treatment visit. For example, it may be possible to correct an airway complication such as obstruction by recognizing labored breathing or sternal retraction even before the patient's oxygen saturation drops. Appropriately assessing the patient's physical state is equally critical before discharge. A patient with excessive drowsiness, instability, and altered gait should continue to be monitored in the office.

Equipment and Mechanical Monitors

- Blood pressure cuff (sphygmomanometer): Blood pressure should be assessed before sedation and before discharge.
- Heart rate/pulse oximeter monitor: Heart rate and blood oxygen saturation should be monitored every 5 minutes throughout the procedure.
- Prechordial stethoscope: A microphone affixed to the patient's suprasternal notch is very useful in detecting respiratory alteration or distress.
- Capnography: A capnograph monitors expired carbon dioxide. This monitor is not currently required per AAPD guidelines, but it has been suggested.

DRUGS FOR PROCEDURAL SEDATION IN PEDIATRIC DENTISTRY

Depending on practitioner experience and training, several medications may be used alone or in combination with other sedatives. Caution should be exercised with administration of multiple agents, as the potential for adverse events increases when drugs are used in combination.[52] When combinations of drugs are used the effect may be synergistic, and the relative doses of each individual medication should be decreased accordingly. Drug classifications for which there is a reversal agent (benzodiazepines, narcotics) should be considered, as the sedative effect may be reversed in the event of oversedation.

Drug Selection

Good sedation practice is to match the patient and procedure with the technique and agent(s) that afford the safest, most humane, and most compassionate care possible. The lightest degree of sedation and analgesia required to achieve this state should be sought.[42] For instance, children with more "difficult" temperament often require higher dosing or administration of multiple agents to produce adequate sedation. Guidance for selection of drug regimen:

- Minimal treatment or short procedure
  - Single agent, with or without nitrous oxide, may be appropriate
  - Example: quick extractions or simple restoration
- Moderate treatment or medium-length procedure
  - Single agent with nitrous oxide may be adequate, but additional agent(s) may be helpful
  - Example: one quadrant of restorative treatment
- Extensive treatment or lengthy procedure
  - Single agent with nitrous oxide may be adequate, but additional agent(s) may be necessary to ensure cooperation and patient comfort
  - Example: multiple quadrants and/or multiple extractions
  - Alternative: divide care into multiple shorter visits and use the "moderate regimen" described above

PREOPERATIVE GUIDELINES

A systematic approach to sedation is a key factor in patient safety. Following a fixed routine and protocol minimizes the potential for human error and the occurrence of adverse events.

Preparation for the Procedure

Instructions to the patient's parent or caregiver should include:

1. Time to arrive at the office
2. Expected wait period following administration of the medications
3. Presence of 2 adults to accompany the child home following treatment. One must devote his or her entire attention to the child while the other drives
4. Instructions to call the office should the child develop an acute illness or changes to their medical status
5. Discussion of NPO instructions (Latin: nil per os, translated nothing by mouth). Preoperative fasting helps ensure that the patient arrives with an empty stomach, thus minimizing chances for emesis and subsequent aspiration, and maximizing absorption of the drug. However, this does leave patients with a greater chance of postoperative dehydration and hypoglycemia (**Table 4**)
6. Instructions to rest with immediate adult supervision for the remainder of the day following sedation

Table 4	
Appropriate intake of food and liquids before elective sedation	
Ingested Material	**Minimum Fasting Period (h)**
Clear liquids: water, fruit juices without pulp, carbonated beverages, clear tea, black coffee	2
Breast milk	4
Infant formula	6
Nonhuman milk: because nonhuman milk is similar to solids in gastric emptying time, the amount ingested must be considered when determining an appropriate fasting period	6
Light meal: a light meal typically consists of toast and clear liquids. Meals that include fried or fatty foods or meat may prolong gastric emptying time. Both the amount and type of foods ingested must be considered when determining an appropriate fasting period.	6

Data from Practice guidelines for preoperative fasting and the use of pharmacologic agents to reduce the risk of pulmonary aspiration: application to healthy patients undergoing elective procedures: an updated report by the American Society of Anesthesiologists Committee on Standards and Practice Parameters. Anesthesiology 2011;114(3):495–511.

7. Discussion of the medication regimen that is planned, including possible side effects and complications

SEDATION PROTOCOL

- Reevaluate the patient's physical status before medication administration. If patients do not meet presedation criteria, the practitioner must be prepared to cancel the case.
- Review the medical history, medications, and allergies.
- Confirm NPO status.
- Document the reason for sedation.
- Discuss the treatment to be provided with the parent.
- Sign and witness the consent form.
- Prepare medications.
  - Confirm with the parent that the child will take oral medication and whether administration is preferred via a cup or oral syringe.
  - Calculate medication dose based on the patient's weight.
  - Retrieve medications from a locked and monitored storage cabinet, in accordance with state and federal regulations. Be familiar with the preparation and appearance of the various medications, as it is easy to become confused if these are varied. It may be safer to use smaller-volume containers (ie, unit-dose preparation) and dispose of the waste, thus ensuring that each patient receives no more than the maximum dose present in the unit-dose vial.
- Calculate maximum local anesthetic and reversal-agent dosages.
- Administer medications.
  - Medications should only be administered under the supervision of the dentist or other qualified observer. Sedation agents must never be given at home before an appointment, because this risks oversedation of the child in a location where they cannot be monitored or rescued.[53]
  - Before administration of the medication, confirm you have the correct patient and correct medication.

- The latent period
  - All sedative medications taken via the oral route have a waiting time or "latent period." This period allows for absorption and drug plasma concentrations which provide the desired effect.
  - Patients should be placed in an area where they can be easily observed by the dental team. Parents should be advised that children must be minimally active during this period, so as to avoid any risk of falling owing to unsteady balance.
- Transfer to the treatment area
  - Once the latent period has passed, the patient is transferred to the treatment area. Because the child will likely be unsteady on his or her feet, it is advisable that the child is transported in a wheelchair or carried to the treatment area. Some parents will prefer to carry the child to the operatory; however, this may make separation more difficult.
- The settling period
  - Moving the child from the waiting room to the treatment area may be quite stimulating, causing even children who appear quite sedated to become more alert. Once the child is placed in the dental chair and the monitors are connected, it is advantageous to "settle" them.
  - The settling period involves placing the nitrous oxide hood on the child's face and instructing him or her to breathe deeply. A high concentration of nitrous oxide (>50%) will intensify the sedative effect.
  - It is important to wait at least 5 minutes for this effect to be fully realized before beginning treatment.
  - Reducing the nitrous oxide concentration after administration of local anesthetic will help avoid higher incidences of nausea and feelings of disorientation and lightheadedness.
  - Minimizing distractions and activity within the room will help calm the child and promote an environment conducive to relaxation.
  - The use of protective stabilization is at the discretion of the provider, but precautions should always be taken to ensure that a sedated child not fall from the chair. Laying children in the stabilization wrap and loosely fastening the legs of the device provides an effective "safety belt."
- Treatment
  - Follow a treatment sequence but be willing to deviate from the plan should behavior deteriorate. Prioritize treatment, completing the most critical items first, thus ensuring that they are completed should the sedative working time expire.
  - Once the child is adequately settled, place topical anesthetic and administer local anesthetic. It is prudent to administer all anesthetic at this time. Injections may be one of the most stimulating portions of the treatment, thus repeating them later in the procedure may prove excessively stimulating, disrupting the sedative effect.
  - Exercise caution in the care of the oral cavity, as protective reflexes are impaired. Patient secretions, water spray, and foreign bodies (stainless-steel crowns, extracted teeth, loose teeth, and so forth) must be taken into account. Limiting use of water and using a rubber dam dramatically decreases the chances of aspiration.
- Postoperative care
  - It is the responsibility of the dental provider to return the child to a state at which safe discharge is possible. A first critical step is to obtain and record postoperative vital signs.

- ○ Assess the patient's level of alertness. If the patient is sufficiently awake, he or she can be given a box of juice or a popsicle, which will help in rehydration and decrease the likelihood of hypoglycemia.
- ○ Before discharge, patients should be ambulatory with assistance, ensuring adequate muscle tone so that they can maintain their own head position. It has been suggested that this can be effectively accomplished if the child meets 2 criteria:
  - Score of 0 or 1 on the University of Michigan Sedation Scale (**Table 5**)
  - Pass the Modified Maintenance of Wakefulness Test during which the child remains awake in a darkened calm environment for 20 minutes[53,54]

COMPLICATIONS

A primary rule of care is primum nonnocere: first do no harm.[42] Thus the cornerstone of safety is prevention of harm. The first key to prevention is obtaining adequate training. The practitioner must master sedation skills from both a theoretical and a practical standpoint. A pediatric dentistry residency is the most traditional means to accomplish this. In such a program, residents complete a GA rotation whereby they become competent in managing the unconscious airway, the gold standard for airway management. It is also possible to obtain or hone skills in airway management through continuing education courses that focus on emergency drills and airway-management simulators.

The second key to prevention is preparedness. The office that practices sedation must possess an up-to-date emergency kit containing emergency drugs (including reversal agents), backup items, and an airway kit that enables them to deliver oxygen under positive pressure. Oxygen is the first line of defense in a sedation emergency, and all members of the team should understand how to administer it to a patient. The dental team should practice emergency drills regularly. Simply planning to call 911 is not an adequate emergency plan; the team should be prepared to rescue the child.

Closed case studies of medical emergencies arising from sedation have consistently indicated that:

- All classes of drugs (sedatives, barbiturates, benzodiazepines, and narcotics) have caused problems, even when administered in the recommended doses.
- Children 1 to 5 years of age are at highest risk. Most had no severe underlying disease.
- Respiratory depression, obstruction, and apnea are the most frequent causes of adverse events. Cardiac and neurologic events are uncommon in healthy children, and these are almost always preceded by a respiratory event.

Table 5	
University of Michigan Sedation Scale	
Score	**Descriptors**
0	Awake and alert
1	Minimally sedated: tired/sleepy, appropriate response to verbal conversation and/or sound
2	Moderately sedated: somnolent/sleeping, easily aroused with light tactile stimulation or a simple verbal command
3	Deeply sedated: deep sleep, arousable only with significant physical stimulation
4	Unarousable

- Adverse events often involved multiple drugs (especially 3 or more sedating medications).
- Basic system-related recommendations and guidelines were often ignored. Drug errors or overdoses, inadequate evaluation, prescription or transcription errors, inadequate monitoring, inadequate resuscitation skills, and premature discharge were involved in adverse effects.
- Most complications from sedation were avoidable.[16,17,19,52,55]

FAILED ATTEMPTS IN PEDIATRIC PROCEDURAL SEDATION

Inadequate levels of sedation and failure to accomplish planned procedures is frustrating to the parent, the patient, and the dental staff. Financial loss from failed sedation attempts may also be quite discouraging; however, the goal of financial success must not supersede what is most prudent or best for patients. Attempting treatment on an unruly, partially sedated patient can compromise patient safety, anger parents, and create stress within the dental team. There is also a substantial medical-legal liability in treating without the parent's consent. When these situations occur, the dentist should admit that treatment has failed and focus on the protection of the child's healthy psyche.

Common reasons why pediatric procedural sedation fails include:

- Poor patient selection, which is the most common reason for failure. GA or perhaps deferred treatment are good alternatives.
- Incorrect medication regimen: A single agent may be inadequate to accomplish quadrant or multiple quadrant dentistry. Use of multiple agents may improve the likelihood of success.
- Unreasonable treatment goals: Attempting to get too much accomplished given the patient, medication, and time available may be a cause for failure. Reasonable treatment goals should be set.
- Inadequate patient preparation: Positive interaction with the child, including adequate explanation of procedures in a language that he or she understands, increases the chances of success.
- Inadequate office preparation: It is important to ensure that the parent understands the financial implications of the procedure when informed consent is obtained. Allowing adequate time in the schedule, and having the proper medications, materials, and functional equipment is also critical to smooth work flow.
- Inadequate or excessive latent period: It is important to be familiar with the medications chosen, allowing for an adequate latent period. Too often dentists have not waited long enough for the medication to have an effect. It is also possible to miss the "window of opportunity" by waiting too long. Educating staff will help increase chances of staying on schedule.
- Wrong time of day: Most children are more cooperative if they are well rested at the time of the visit. On occasion, it may be necessary to sedate a child in the afternoon. Following NPO guidelines by allowing clear liquids until up to 2 hours before arrival and having a nap may improve the child's ability to endure an afternoon procedure.
- Incorrect dosage or medication: Familiarity with medications decreases chances for error. A common reason for error is interruption while drawing medications. If you believe that you may have dispensed the wrong dosage or medication, a good rule of thumb is "when in doubt, throw it out."

- Excessively stimulating treatment environment: It is best to use a quiet room with lower volume of ambient noise. Dimming the lights may help calm a child. Place sharp or threatening dental instruments out of sight of the child, and remember that patients observe the environment around them. Encourage the child to bring a special toy, stuffed animal, or blanket if it will make him or her feel more secure.

SUMMARY

For children who are young, anxious, or have extensive treatment needs, procedural sedation may be a safe, effective, and humane way to facilitate delivery of dental care. Sedation should only be provided by practitioners who are adequately trained and understand indications, contraindications, agent(s), dosage, adverse effects, and rescue techniques. Successful outcomes depend on a systematic approach to care, including adequate presedation and postsedation evaluation, following appropriate monitoring and equipment guidelines, and having the knowledge and skills to manage adverse cardiopulmonary events.

REFERENCES

1. Wilson S, Nathan JE. A survey study of sedation training in advanced pediatric dentistry programs: thoughts of program directors and students. Pediatr Dent 2011;33(4):353–60.
2. Houpt M. Project USAP the use of sedative agents in pediatric dentistry: 1991 update. Pediatr Dent 1993;15(1):36–40.
3. Houpt MI. Project USAP—part III: practice by heavy users of sedation in pediatric dentistry. ASDC J Dent Child 1993;60(3):183–5.
4. Houpt M. Project USAP 2000—use of sedative agents by pediatric dentists: a 15-year follow-up survey. Pediatr Dent 2002;24(4):289–94.
5. Casamassimo PS, Wilson S, Gross L. Effects of changing U.S. parenting styles on dental practice: perceptions of diplomates of the American Board of Pediatric Dentistry presented to the College of Diplomates of the American Board of Pediatric Dentistry 16th Annual Session, Atlanta, GA, Saturday, May 26, 2001. Pediatr Dent 2002;24(1):18–22.
6. Wilson S. Pharmacological management of the pediatric dental patient. Pediatr Dent 2004;26(2):131–6.
7. American Academy of Pediatrics Committee on Drugs: guidelines for monitoring and management of pediatric patients during and after sedation for diagnostic and therapeutic procedures. Pediatrics 1992;89(6 Pt 1):1110–5.
8. Guidelines for monitoring and management of pediatric patients during and after sedation for diagnostic and therapeutic procedures: addendum. Pediatrics 2002; 110(4):836–8.
9. Adair SM. Evidence-based use of fluoride in contemporary pediatric dental practice. Pediatr Dent 2006;28(2):133–42 [discussion: 92–8].
10. Amin MS, Harrison RL, Benton TS, et al. Effect of povidone-iodine on *Streptococcus mutans* in children with extensive dental caries. Pediatr Dent 2004; 26(1):5–10.
11. Simratvir M, Singh N, Chopra S, et al. Efficacy of 10% povidone iodine in children affected with early childhood caries: an in vivo study. J Clin Pediatr Dent 2010; 34(3):233–8.
12. Zhan L, Featherstone JD, Gansky SA, et al. Antibacterial treatment needed for severe early childhood caries. J Public Health Dent 2006;66(3):174–9.

13. American Academy of Pediatric Dentistry Council on Clinical Affairs. Policy on interim therapeutic restorations (ITR). Pediatr Dent 2008;30(Suppl 7):38–9.

14. Lee J, Vann W, Roberts M. A cost analysis of treating pediatric dental patients using general anesthesia versus conscious sedation. Pediatr Dent 2000;22:27–32.

15. Boyle CA. Sedation or general anaesthesia for treating anxious children. Evid Based Dent 2009;10(3):69.

16. Kaplan RF, Yang CI. Sedation and analgesia in pediatric patients for procedures outside the operating room. Anesthesiol Clin North America 2002;20(1):181–94, vii.

17. Guideline for monitoring and management of pediatric patients during and after sedation for diagnostic and therapeutic procedures. Pediatr Dent 2008; 30(Suppl 7):143–59.

18. American Academy of Pediatric Dentistry Clinical Affairs Committee. Guideline on behavior guidance for the pediatric dental patient; 2011. p. 161–73.

19. Cote CJ. "Conscious sedation": time for this oxymoron to go away! J Pediatr 2001;139:15–7 [discussion: 18–9].

20. Wilkinson GR. Drug metabolism and variability among patients in drug response. N Engl J Med 2005;352:2211–21.

21. Doyle L, Colletti JE. Pediatric procedural sedation and analgesia. Pediatr Clin North Am 2006;53:279–92.

22. JCAHO. Comprehensive accreditation manual for hospitals. Oakbrook (IL); 2000.

23. JCAHO. Revisions to anesthesia care standards. Comprehensive Accreditation Manual for Ambulatory Care; 2012.

24. Lourenco-Matharu L, Ashley PF, Furness S. Sedation of children undergoing dental treatment. Cochrane Database Syst Rev 2012;(3):CD003877.

25. Ashley PF, Williams CE, Moles DR, et al. Sedation versus general anaesthesia for provision of dental treatment in under 18 year olds. Cochrane Database Syst Rev 2009;(1):CD006334.

26. Jensen B, Stjernqvist K. Temperament and acceptance of dental treatment under sedation in preschool children. Acta Odontol Scand 2002;60(4):231–6.

27. Fraone G, Wilson S, Casamassimo PS, et al. The effect of orally administered midazolam on children of three age groups during restorative dental care. Pediatr Dent 1999;21(4):235–41.

28. Quinonez R, Santos RG, Boyar R, et al. Temperament and trait anxiety as predictors of child behavior prior to general anesthesia for dental surgery. Pediatr Dent 1997;19(6):427–31.

29. Lochary ME, Wilson S, Griffen AL, et al. Temperament as a predictor of behavior for conscious sedation in dentistry. Pediatr Dent 1993;15(5):348–52.

30. Radis FG, Wilson S, Griffen AL, et al. Temperament as a predictor of behavior during initial dental examination in children. Pediatr Dent 1994;16(2):121–7.

31. Voepel-Lewis T, Malviya S, Prochaska G, et al. Sedation failures in children undergoing MRI and CT: is temperament a factor? Paediatr Anaesth 2000;10(3): 319–23.

32. Cohen LL, Francher A, MacLaren JE, et al. Correlates of pediatric behavior and distress during intramuscular injections for invasive dental procedures. J Clin Pediatr Dent 2006;31(1):44–7.

33. Arnrup K, Broberg AG, Berggren U, et al. Lack of cooperation in pediatric dentistry—the role of child personality characteristics. Pediatr Dent 2002;24(2): 119–28.

34. Arnrup K, Berggren U, Broberg AG, et al. A short-term follow-up of treatment outcome in groups of uncooperative child dental patients. Eur J Paediatr Dent 2004;5(4):216–24.

35. de Oliveira VJ, da Costa LR, Marcelo VC, et al. Mothers' perceptions of children's refusal to undergo dental treatment: an exploratory qualitative study. Eur J Oral Sci 2006;114(6):471–7.
36. American Society of Anesthesiologists. ASA relative value guide: ASA physical status classification system. American Society of Anesthesiologists; 2011.
37. Jackson DL, Johnson BS. Conscious sedation for dentistry: risk management and patient selection. Dent Clin North Am 2002;46(4):767–80.
38. Aplin S, Baines D, DE Lima J. Use of the ASA Physical Status Grading System in pediatric practice. Paediatr Anaesth 2007;17:216–22.
39. Cohen MM, Cameron CB. Should you cancel the operation when a child has an upper respiratory tract infection? Anesth Analg 1991;72(3):282–8.
40. Olsson GL, Hallen B. Laryngospasm during anaesthesia. A computer-aided incidence study in 136,929 patients. Acta Anaesthesiol Scand 1984;28(5):567–75.
41. Schreiner MS, O'Hara I, Markakis DA, et al. Do children who experience laryngospasm have an increased risk of upper respiratory tract infection? Anesthesiology 1996;85(3):475–80.
42. Rodriguez E, Jordan R. Contemporary trends in pediatric sedation and analgesia. Emerg Med Clin North Am 2002;20(1):199–222.
43. Krauss B, Green SM. Procedural sedation and analgesia in children. Lancet 2006;367:766–80.
44. Malviya S, D'Errico C, Reynolds P, et al. Should pregnancy testing be routine in adolescent patients prior to surgery? Anesth Analg 1996;83(4):854–8.
45. Wheeler M, Cote CJ. Preoperative pregnancy testing in a tertiary care children's hospital: a medico-legal conundrum. J Clin Anesth 1999;11:56–63.
46. American Dental Association Council on Access, Prevention and Interprofessional Relations. Women's oral health issues. American Dental Association; 2006.
47. Ang-Lee MK, Moss J, Yuan CS. Herbal medicines and perioperative care. JAMA 2001;286:208–16.
48. Culver JL, Walker JR. Anesthetic implications of illicit drug use. J Perianesth Nurs 1999;14:82–90.
49. Hyatt B, Bensky KP. Illicit drugs and anesthesia. CRNA 1999;10(1):15–23.
50. Fishbaugh DF, Wilson S, Preisch JW, et al. Relationship of tonsil size on an airway blockage maneuver in children during sedation. Pediatr Dent 1997;19(4):277–81.
51. Chan J, Edman JC, Koltai PJ. Obstructive sleep apnea in children. Am Fam Physician 2004;69(5):1147–54.
52. Cote CJ, Notterman DA, Karl HW, et al. Adverse sedation events in pediatrics: a critical incident analysis of contributing factors. Pediatrics 2000;105(4 Pt 1):805–14.
53. Cote CJ. Discharge criteria for children sedated by nonanesthesiologists: is "safe" really safe enough? Anesthesiology 2004;100:207–9.
54. Malviya S, Voepel-Lewis T, Ludomirsky A, et al. Can we improve the assessment of discharge readiness?: a comparative study of observational and objective measures of depth of sedation in children. Anesthesiology 2004;100:218–24.
55. Practice guidelines for sedation and analgesia by non-anesthesiologists. Anesthesiology 2002;96(4):1004–17.

Providing Dental Treatment for Children in a Hospital Setting

Elizabeth Velan, DMD, MSD[a,*], Barbara Sheller, DDS, MSD[a,b]

KEYWORDS

- Dental hospital care • Operating room • Special health care needs

KEY POINTS

- To promote oral health for an ever-increasing number of patients with special health care needs (SHCNs), all dentists have a role.
- It is not possible for pediatric dentists to see every patient with special needs throughout their lifetime.
- General dental practices and community clinics are the foundation of dental health care in the United States.
- It is important to train general dentists to care for medically and behaviorally complex patients, to encourage them to seek hospital privileging, including care in operating rooms (ORs), and to support hospital dental programs.

INTRODUCTION

Hospital-based dentistry is a rewarding way to contribute to the community and add variety to a pediatric or general dental practice. Hospital training is a requirement in all accredited pediatric dental and general dental residency programs.[1,2] Once certification is completed, however, many dentists never return to the hospital to provide patient care. This article presents information about providing dental treatment in a hospital. The primary focus is providing dental treatment in a hospital OR. Hospital outpatient dental clinics, inpatient dental consultations, and dental treatment in emergency departments are discussed briefly.

National data demonstrate that the number of children and adults with SHCNs is growing. This increase can be attributed to improvements in medical and surgical care because conditions that were once fatal have become chronic and manageable

[a] Department of Pediatric Dentistry, Seattle Children's Hospital, School of Dentistry, University of Washington, 4800 Sandpoint Way NE, Seattle, WA 98105, USA; [b] Department of Orthodontics, Seattle Children's Hospital, School of Dentistry, University of Washington, 1959 NE Pacific St, Seattle, WA 98195, USA
* Corresponding author.
E-mail address: Elizabeth.velan@seattlechildrens.org

Dent Clin N Am 57 (2013) 163–173
http://dx.doi.org/10.1016/j.cden.2012.09.003
0011-8532/13/$ – see front matter © 2013 Elsevier Inc. All rights reserved.

dental.theclinics.com

problems. Concurrently, societal changes have brought inclusiveness to individuals with developmental disabilities; rarely is a child institutionalized for Down syndrome or autism. The percentage of households with children in the United States with 1 or more children with SHCNs increased from 22% to 28% between 2001 and 2008.[3]

Health care for some individuals with SHCNs requires specialized knowledge, increased awareness and attention, and adaptation and accommodative measures beyond what is considered routine.[4] Most patients with SHCNs receive dental care in their community; for a subset of these patients, definitive dental care in a hospital OR or clinic may be the best treatment option.

There are several differences between dental practice within a hospital versus in a clinic or private office. Most differences are due to accreditations and regulations. Hospitals are accredited by The Joint Commission (TJC). Thus, an accredited hospital must follow standards set by TJC. All providers practicing in a hospital must join the hospital professional staff and have hospital privileges, which are specific permissions relating to the area of practice and that meet documentation standards set by TJC.

PATIENT SELECTION FOR DENTAL CARE IN HOSPITALS

Most patients who receive dental treatment in hospitals have SHCNs. A 2010 survey of a hospital outpatient dental clinic found most patients presented with either medical complexity or intellectual/behavioral limitations that prevented their cooperation for dental procedures.[5] For uncooperative patients with SHCNs, dentists may use a continuum of behavior guidance strategies, ranging from simple communicative techniques to oral or parenteral sedation. Pediatric dentists and dentists treating adults with SHCNs have embraced the concept of in-office general anesthesia (GA) for dental treatment where GA is provided by a medical or dental anesthesiologist or by a certified nurse anesthetist, depending on practitioner availability and state practice requirements.[6–8]

In-office sedation or GA may be unsafe for patients with complex medical conditions and/or severe behavioral limitations. Hospital or university-based dental clinics may be the only venue for these patients to receive care. Clinics that serve this population are not widely available and are not distributed evenly across the United States.[9,10] For families needing to seek care at these institutions, travel and long wait times can be expected. For adults with SHCNs, dental care may be difficult to access. A study of oral health status of adults with intellectual and developmental disabilities receiving dental care in Massachusetts through state-supported clinics in 2009–2010 found prevalence of periodontal disease was 80% and untreated caries was 32%.[11] A 2012 survey in New York found a 1-year to 2-year wait for dental services in the OR for adults with SHCNs.[12]

Because capacity in hospital dental clinics is limited, they should be reserved for those who cannot be safely treated in the community. Offering a dental home to patients with SHCNs in private dental practices and community clinics for preventive/recall services with the back-up of taking patients with significant treatment needs to the OR is the best way to accommodate the increasing population of patients with SHCNs.

PLANNING DENTAL CARE UNDER GENERAL ANESTHESIA IN A HOSPITAL OPERATING ROOM

A comprehensive dental examination, pending behavioral constraints, should be completed to assess treatment needs, such as restorations, exodontia, and periodontal or endodontic procedures, before care under GA is considered. If there are minimal dental needs, the risks of GA do not outweigh the benefits. The American Society of Anesthesiologists risk assessment classification (ASA class) is often used to assess anesthesia risk and to determine the appropriate venue for GA (**Table 1**).[13] The risk of anesthesia increases with higher ASA status and with certain types of surgical procedures. Dental procedures are generally considered low risk. Risk of GA for patients with SHCNs undergoing dental procedures is presumed higher than in healthy peers but has not been adequately studied.[14] Nearly all ASA class I and mild ASA class II patients can be treated safely with in-office GA.

Most patients receiving care in a hospital OR have ASA classification II or III. An example of an ASA II patient appropriate for a hospital setting is a large teenage patient with violent behaviors related to autism. In a hospital, there is sufficient staff to assist with the unpredictable recovery of such a patient. ASA III and IV patients should have care in the hospital (**Table 2**). It is important to work closely with anesthesia providers and be acquainted with their practice philosophy. Many hospitals offer an anesthesia consultation for patients before the day of surgery. Some patients may be acceptable risks only for anesthesiologists practicing in tertiary-care centers.

Dentists can approximate a patient's ASA classification by taking a comprehensive medical history (**Table 3**).[15] Ambiguous information should be clarified by a discussion with the primary care physician or medical specialist. Additional information needed when planning GA is a history of adverse reaction to GA by the patient or a family member.

The dental examination should identify patients with potentially complex airways. Conditions of concern are limited neck mobility, cervical spine instability, severely retrusive maxilla, micrognathic mandible, limited jaw opening, and macroglossia.[16] If a patient is cooperative, the tongue should be rated using the Mallampati classification (**Fig. 1**). For this examination, the patient is seated with head in a neutral position, the mouth is opened, and the tongue protruded as far as possible (**Table 4**).[17] Patients with Mallampati classification 3 or 4 are more likely to have difficult airways.

Patients with SHCNs may have needs for other surgical or diagnostic services in addition to dental treatment. In some cases, procedures can be combined under a single GA. A 2007 study in a pediatric hospital found the procedures most commonly combined with dentistry were oral surgery, otolaryngology, and brainstem auditory evoked response heath (BAER) test.[18] Many surgical procedures are not appropriate to do simultaneously with dental treatment; examples are placing central lines, neurologic procedures, and most orthopedic procedures. If considering combination care, an early call to the other surgeon or proceduralist determines if combination is feasible.

A postsurgery recovery plan should be made at the examination appointment. A majority of patients with SHCNs are discharged to home within hours after dental surgery. Any patient unlikely to meet postanesthesia discharge requirements should

Table 1	
American Society of Anesthesiologists risk assessment classification	
Class I	A normally healthy patient with no organic, physiologic, biologic, biochemical, or psychiatric disturbance or disease
Class II	A patient with mild-to-moderate systemic disturbance or disease
Class III	A patient with severe systemic disturbance or disease
Class IV	A patient with severe and life-threatening systemic disease or disorder
Class V	A moribund patient who is unlikely to survive without the planned procedure
Class VI	A declared brain dead patient whose organs are being removed for donor purposes

Table 2
Examples of ASA classification

ASA II	ASA III	ASA IV
Well-controlled asthma	Difficult to control asthma, diabetes, seizure disorder	Unrepaired cyanotic heart disease
Well-controlled diabetes	Autism with comorbidity, such as seizure disorder	Advanced progressive disease
Well-controlled hypertension	Down syndrome with severe comorbidity, such as	• Spinal muscular atrophy
Corrected arterio or ventricular septal defects with no residual disease	• Antlantoaxial instability	• Muscular dystrophy
Autism	• Repaired tetralogy of Fallot	• Cystic fibrosis
Stable mental health disease	Unrepaired congenital heart defect	
Pregnant	Tracheostomy status	
	Cancer in active treatment	

Table 3
Medical history

General	Name, date of birth Legal guardian and phone number Height, weight, body mass index Name and phone number of physicians
Medications	Name and dose, include over the counter and supplements
Allergies	Drugs, food, and environmental, include reaction
Hospitalizations	Reason, date, and outcome
Surgeries	Reason, date, and outcome
Birth history	Complications during pregnancy and/or birth, prematurity
Genetic disorders	Name, date diagnosed
Head	Ears, eyes, nose, and throat
Cardiovascular	Congenital heart defect/disease, heart murmur, high blood pressure
Respiratory	Asthma, reactive airway disease/breathing problems, smoking (including second-hand smoke), chronic lung disease, infectious disease of lungs
Gastrointestinal	Eating disorder, ulcer, gastroesophageal reflux disease, chronic or transient infections of liver, gastrostomy tube, failure to thrive
Genitourinary	Kidney disease
Musculoskeletal	Arthritis, scoliosis, joint replacement
Neurologic	Seizure disorder, neuromuscular disease
Hematologic	Anemia, bleeding disorders, history of blood transfusions, cancer treatment or history of
Immunologic	Immunocompromised
Behavior	Personality: easy, shy, difficult Developmental or intellectual disabilities Mental health problems
Social	Travel constraints Dysfunctional social situation/difficulty with continuity of care

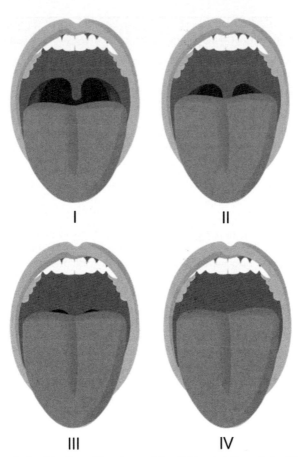

Fig. 1. Mallampati classification. (*Courtesy of* Jordi March i Nogué, La Bisbal d'Empordà, Spain. Available at: http://en.wikipedia.org/wiki/Mallampati_classification; with permission.)

be planned for admission to the hospital for extended observation. **Box 1** gives examples of conditions that often result in admission after dental care under GA (B. Sheller, DDS, MSD, personal communication, 2012).[19] Infrequently, patients are admitted postoperatively due to long-distance travel for care and/or questionable ability of caretakers to comply with postoperative instructions. In many hospitals, a medical hospitalist service exists to manage patient medical problems during surgical recovery. Verify requirements for handing off a patient for admission when dental treatment is completed at a hospital. **Fig. 2** presents a decision tree for selecting a venue for dental treatment under GA.

Table 4 Mallampati classification	
Class 1	Visualization of the soft palate, fauces, uvula, and anterior and posterior pillars
Class 2	Visualization of the soft palate, fauces, and uvula
Class 3	Visualization of the soft palate and base of the uvula
Class 4	Soft palate not visible

Box 1
Patients who may need to be admitted for observation after dental procedure

- Patients with severe obstructive sleep apnea requiring a bilevel positive airway pressure or continuous positive airway pressure
- Patients not expected to maintain nutritional intake
- Patients with severe bleeding disorders
- Patients with cyanotic heart disease with compensatory hemodynamics
- Patients with difficultly with oral secretions, high aspiration risk
- Patients with severe restrictive lung disease
- Patients expected to need blood products soon after surgical procedure (pre-existing medical condition)

Dentists may want to prepare a patient information handout about receiving treatment at a hospital OR that includes contact numbers, items for the patient to complete in advance of surgery, and expectations for the day, including restrictions on eating and drinking (nothing by mouth requirement).

COUNTDOWN TO SURGERY

All hospitals accredited by TJC require a history and physical (H&P) examination (**Table 5**)[15] to be completed within 30 days of the surgery date. At the time of the dental

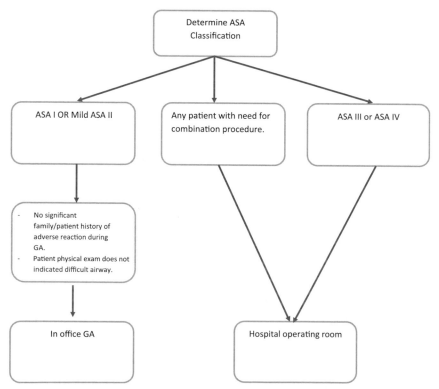

Fig. 2. Flow chart for determining venue for dental treatment under anesthesia.

Table 5 History and physical examination	
Constitutional	Height–weight–body mass index–SaO_2–temperature Pulse/rate and rhythm Blood pressure General body habitus
Ears, nose, mouth, and throat	Tympanic membrane Mucosa of nose and oral cavity Gingiva and tongue Tonsils and pharynx
Eyes	Conjunctiva–lids–pupils/iris No foreign body
Neck	Range of motion Thyroid gland
Lymphatic	Location–enlargement–tenderness–symmetry
Gastrointestinal	Bowel sounds–masses–hepatosplenomegaly Perianal area without masses or tenderness
Skin	Integrity Temperature
Breasts	No masses or tenderness
Musculoskeletal	Clubbing, digital pallor, or cyanosis Alignment, symmetry, range of motion Normal digital sensation/circulation
Respiratory	Chest shape Clear to auscultation Symmetric breath sounds Stridor–wheezing–grunting–flaring/retracting
Genitourinary	Kidney disease
Cardiac	Murmur–gallop–rub–thrill Radial pulse, capillary refill time Pulse in groin–pedal pulse Edema
Neurologic/psychological	Alert/oriented Cooperative for age Cranial nerves II–XII intact Cerebellar: gait–coordination–balance Strength/tone Sensation grossly intact Cognition normal for age: memory–language–development Mood/affect

examination, inform the family about the H&P protocol. The hospital may require use of a standard H&P form. An anesthesiology consultation within a month of surgery allows identification of any medical issues or indication for laboratory testing to be resolved before the date of surgery.

SAMPLE DAY AT THE HOSPITAL

The patient experience at the hospital is divided into preoperative, operative and post-operative phases (**Boxes 2** and **3**). Preoperative check-in at the authors' institution begins 90 minutes before the surgical start time. The surgery start time is generally determined by the hospital considering length of surgical procedure, patient age, and medical status.

Box 2
Preoperative phase

- Family checks in
- Family is brought to preinduction room
- Nurse completes institutional dependent preoperative forms, including nothing by mouth status, weight, height, pain score, medications, and drug allergies
- Surgeon completes/reviews consent and answers questions
- Surgeon confirms H&P (within 30 days of procedure)
- Family meets anesthesia team and answers questions
- Premed given (if indicated) by anesthesia team; IV may be placed
- Circulating nurse meets patient answers questions, confirmation of completed forms
- Anesthesia provider and nurse complete final safety check and bring patient to OR for induction

---

The operative phase begins when a patient enters the OR or anesthesia induction room. After induction of anesthesia and intubation, a time out is conducted with the entire surgical team. All team concerns should be discussed and resolved before the initiation of the surgical procedure. The patient is appropriately padded and positioned. All OR personnel must follow Occupational Safety and Health Administration guidelines, including OR attire, hand hygiene, and use of personal protective equipment. Dental equipment used in the OR is the same as that is used in a dental clinic. The dentist must be mindful that a patient's protective reflexes are removed by GA and continual attention is needed to protect oral soft tissues during treatment. When dental treatment is finished, institution-dependent documentation is completed, which may include a brief operative note, postoperative orders, and a surgery team sign out. Extubation and transfer of the patient to the PACU ends the operative phase. **Box 3** summarizes the operative phase.

In the PACU, the patient's vital signs are monitored and treatment is given as needed for pain or emesis. Parameters monitored are (1) respiratory: rate, airway patency, and oxygen saturation; (2) cardiovascular: pulse and blood pressure; (3) neuromuscular; and (4) mental status.[20] Once patients are awake and stable, they are transferred to phase II recovery or admitted to a medical hospitalist service. Pending hospital procedures and type of anesthesia, some patients may be fast-tracked directly from the OR to phase II recovery.[21] Patients must meet hospital discharge criteria before release from the hospital.

Dentist responsibilities postoperatively include dictating an operative report, writing prescriptions for discharge medications, communication with the hospitalist for patients being admitted, and having a postoperative discussion with patient caregivers. Written postoperative instructions should include suggestions for liquids and foods, pain management plan, oral hygiene, care for extraction or periodontal surgery, and 24/7 contact numbers in the event of patient difficulty after discharge. Depending on the dental treatment provided, a postoperative appointment may be needed.

ESTABLISHING PRIVILEGES

Once a decision has been made to participate in a hospital setting, dentists must seek privileges. Some basic requirements for medical staff membership and hospital

---

Box 3
Operative phase

- Intubation completed by anesthesia team
  - Nasoendotracheal tube preferred or oral RAE if nasoendotracheal not possible
  - Airway is secured
  - Eye protection placed
  - Turban placed to protect hair and ears
- Time out is completed with entire surgical team
- Antibiotics given (if appropriate)
- Patient is positioned for treatment, head rest, and shoulder roll
- Appropriate padding is completed, Foley catheter (dependent on case time), warming blankets
- Dental procedure started
  - Lead shield placed on patient and OR personnel
  - Radiographs taken
  - Throat pack placed to protect airway, time in recorded
  - Débridement completed followed by a prophylaxis and examination
  - Treatment plan finalized
  - A mouth prop is used to maintain opening with careful placement to avoid damage to soft tissue
  - Rubber dam is used for isolation during restorative treatment (protects soft tissue and prevents debris in airway)
  - Extractions—local anesthetic used for postoperative pain relief and assist with hemostasis type and amount recorded
  - Oral cavity rinsed and suctioned, throat pack is removal, time out recorded
- Postoperative forms completed
- Postoperative medications prescribed
- Postoperative orders completed
- Safety sign out is completed by entire surgical team
- Patient extubated and brought to the postanesthesia care unit (PACU)

---

privileges are graduation from an accredited dental school, a current state license, high ethical and moral standards, and professional liability insurance.[15] The application may ask how many hospital-based dental procedures a dentist has completed during advanced training and require a letter from a graduate program director. Some hospitals may require board certification. Applications for privileges are most readily obtained through a hospital's medical staff office and/or a hospital's Web site. The credentialing process may take several months. Dentists should expect to pay an annual fee and to renew privileges biannually.

Once hospital privileges are obtained, it is important to work only in the area of delineation of privileges. For example, a dentist may have ambulatory privileges only and not be able to see patients admitted to the hospital or may have both. The privileges may be different for outpatient and inpatient components. Timely completion of medical records is expected and there may be a requirement to participate in emergency on-call rotations.

HOSPITAL DENTAL CLINICS, DENTAL CONSULTATION FOR INPATIENTS, AND DENTISTRY IN EMERGENCY DEPARTMENTS

A hospital dental clinic plays a role in the comprehensive care of some patients with SHCNs. Among reasons for establishing a dental home in a hospital clinic are medical complexity, need for coordinated care with medical and dental specialties, and lack of community options. A 2010 survey of more than 900 patients receiving dental care at a pediatric hospital dental clinic found nearly all patients to have SHCNs and concluded that a hospital dental clinic is an appropriate dental home for those children with complex medical conditions, such as cyanotic heart malformations with compensatory hemodynamics, dystrophic epidermolysis bullosa, or end-stage renal disease.[5]

Dentists play an important role in optimal management of certain hospital inpatients. A 2007 study of consultations at a pediatric hospital found consultations were requested most often by hematology/oncology, transplant oncology, pediatric medicine, and rehabilitation medicine. Frequent reasons for consult requests were baseline evaluation, oral pain, to rule-out a dental cause of fever, and managing self-injurious patient behavior.[22]

Hospital emergency departments have become a source of primary care for primary care medicine and dentistry. Although emergency departments are inefficient for management of dental problems, patients without a dental home may not have any other options.[23] If dentists receive hospital privileges, they may be called on to assess and treat patients presenting to an emergency department.

To promote oral health for an ever-increasing number of patients with SHCNs, all dentists have a role. It is not possible for pediatric dentists to see every patient with special needs throughout their lifetime. General dental practices and community clinics are the foundation of dental health care in the United States. It is important to train general dentists to care for medically and behaviorally complex patients, to encourage them to seek hospital privileging including care in ORs, and to support hospital dental programs.

REFERENCES

1. Accreditation standards for advanced Specialty Education programs in pediatric dentistry. Chicago, IL: Commission on Dental Accreditation, American Dental Association; 1998.
2. Accreditation standards for advanced Education programs in general practice residency. Chicago, IL: Commission on Dental Accreditation, American Dental Association; 2007.
3. Available at: http://mchb.hrsa.gov/cshcn05/NF/1prevalence/individual. Accessed July, 2012
4. American Academy of Pediatric Dentistry. Guideline on management of dental patients with special health care needs. Pediatr Dent 2009;32(6):132–6.
5. Mudd D. Outpatient dental services at seattle children's hospital—a descriptive study [MSD Thesis]. Seattle: University of Washington; 2010.
6. Olabi NF, Jones JE, Saxen MA, et al. The use of office-based sedation and general anesthesia by board certified pediatric dentists practicing in the United States. Anesth Prog 2012;59:12–7.
7. American Academy of Pediatric Dentistry. Policy on the use of deep sedation and general anesthesia in the pediatric dental office. Pediatr Dent 2007;32(6):67–8.

8. Tarver M, Guelmann M, Primosch R. Impact of office-based intravenous deep sedation providers upon traditional sedation practices employed in pediatric dentistry. Pediatr Dent 2012;34(3):62–8.
9. Kerins C, Casamassimo PS, Ciesla D, et al. A preliminary analysis of the US dental health care system's capacity to treat children with special health care needs. Pediatr Dent 2011;33(2):107–12.
10. Ciesla D, Kerins CA, Seale NS, et al. Characteristics of dental clinics in US children's hospitals. Pediatr Dent 2011;33(2):100–6.
11. Morgan JP, Minihan PM, Stark PC, et al. The oral health status of 4,732 adults with intellectual and developmental disabilities. J Am Dent Assoc 2012;143:838–46.
12. Tegtmeir CH. Survey of ambulatory surgery dentistry. N Y State Dent J 2012;78: 38–45.
13. Wolters U, Wolf T, Stützer H, et al. ASA classification and perioperative variables as predictors of postoperative outcome. Br J Anaesth 1996;77:217–22.
14. Messieha Z. Risks of general anesthesia for the special needs dental patient. Spec Care Dentist 2009;29(1):21–5.
15. Nowak AJ, Casamassimo PS, editors. The American Academy of Pediatric Dentistry Handbook of Pediatric Dentistry. 4th edition. Chicago, IL; 2011.
16. Petranker S, Levon N, Ogle OE. Preoperative evaluation of the surgical patient. Dent Clin North Am 2012;56:163–81.
17. Mallampati S, Gatt S, Gugino LD, et al. A clinical sign to predict difficult tracheal intubation: a prospective study. Can Anaesth Soc J 1985;32(4):429–34.
18. Stapleton M, Sheller B, Williams BJ, et al. Combining procedures under general anesthesia. Pediatr Dent 2007;29(5):397–402.
19. Biro P, Kaplan V, Block KE. Anesthetic management of a patient with obstructive sleep apnea syndrome and difficult airway access. J Clin Anesth 1995;7:417–21.
20. American Society of Anesthesiologists. Practice guidelines for postanesthetic care. A report by the American Society of Anesthesiologists Task Force on Postanesthetic Care. Anesthesiology 2002;96(3):742–52.
21. White PF, Song F, Song D. New Criteria for fast-tracking after outpatient anesthesia: a comparison with the modified Aldrete's scoring system. Anesth Analg 1999;88:1069–72.
22. Kanuga S, Sheller B, Williams BJ, et al. A one-year survey of inpatient dental consultations at a children's hospital. Spec Care Dentist 2012;32(1):26–31.
23. Rowley ST, Sheller B, Williams BJ, et al. Utilization of a hospital for treatment of pediatric dental emergencies. Pediatr Dent 2006;28(1):10–7.

Index

Note: Page numbers of article titles are in **boldface** type.

A

Ameloblastic fibroma, 92, 93
Ameloblastomas, 90, 91
Anesthesia, and sedation, continuum of, 147–148
   general, for behavioral guidance, 139–140
Arthritis, juvenile idiopathic, and temporomandibular joint disorders, 108, 109
Avulsion, due to trauma, 47–48, 51

B

Behavior guidance, advanced strategies for, 137–140
   age-related psychosocial traits and, 132, 133
   alternative restorative treatments and, 136–137
   audiovisual distraction and, 135
   communicative, 134
   continuum of, **129–143**
   general anesthesia for, 139–140
   nitrous oxide/oxygen inhalation and, 135–136
   parental presence/absence and, 135
   patient assessment for, 132
      medical history in, 132–133
      parent/caregiver preferences and, 134
      pretreatment, 132–134
      temperament evaluation in, 133
   pharmacologic, 147
   principles of, 130–132
   protective stabilization in, 137–138
   sedation in, 138–139, 147
      alternatives to, 147
      goals of, 147
   techniques in, 130
Bone cavity, idiopathic, 90, 91
Bruxism, 105–107
Buccal infected cyst, 90

C

Canines, labially positioned, 28–31
   palatally positioned, 31–33
   unerupted, 28, 31

Dent Clin N Am 57 (2013) 175–180
http://dx.doi.org/10.1016/S0011-8532(12)00107-3
0011-8532/13/$ – see front matter © 2013 Elsevier Inc. All rights reserved.

dental.theclinics.com

Moving?

Make sure your subscription moves with you!

To notify us of your new address, find your **Clinics Account Number** (located on your mailing label above your name), and contact customer service at:

Email: journalscustomerservice-usa@elsevier.com

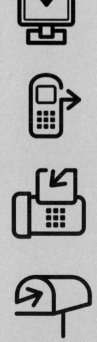

800-654-2452 (subscribers in the U.S. & Canada)
314-447-8871 (subscribers outside of the U.S. & Canada)

Fax number: 314-447-8029

Elsevier Health Sciences Division
Subscription Customer Service
3251 Riverport Lane
Maryland Heights, MO 63043

*To ensure uninterrupted delivery of your subscription, please notify us at least 4 weeks in advance of move.